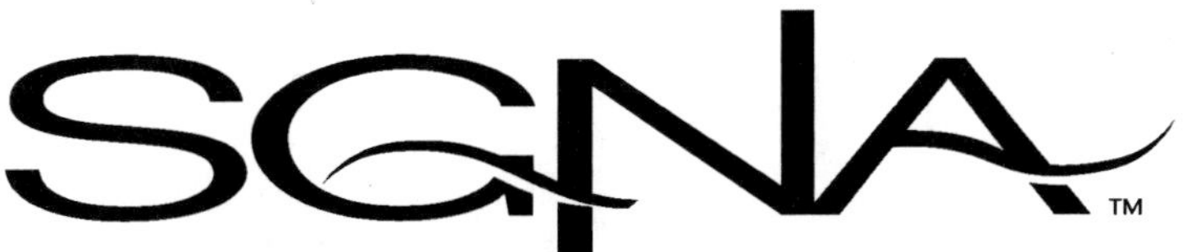

Society of Gastroenterology Nurses and Associates, Inc.

MANUAL OF PULMONARY PROCEDURES FOR ENDOSCOPY NURSES

3rd Edition

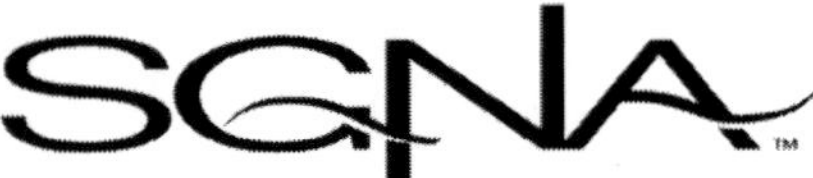

401 North Michigan Avenue
Chicago, IL 60611-4267 USA
Telephone: 312/321-5165 or 800/245-7462
Fax: 312/673-6694
Email: SGNA@smithbucklin.com
www.sgna.org

Printed in the United States of America

First Edition 2001

ISBN 0-9855091-0-4

Table of Contents

Part 4: SAFETY

Part 5: STANDARD EQUIPMENT

APPENDICES

Acknowledgements

Illustrations used in this manual have been provided courtesy of the following:

Bard Endoscopic Technologies
Boston Scientific Microvasive
David Crandall
ERBE USA, Inc.
Sharon Lesser, RN

Disclaimer

The Society of Gastroenterology Nurses and Associates, Inc. presents this manual as an educational treatise for use in developing institutional policies, procedures, and/or protocols specific to the gastrointestinal endoscopy setting. Suggested procedures should be modified based on clinical assessment or the individual needs of each patient.

The Society of Gastroenterology Nurses and Associates, Inc., the contributors, and the reviewers assume no responsibility for any adverse or harmful effects or any liability resulting directly or indirectly from the suggested procedures, from any unknown errors or omissions, from the practitioner's use of the procedure in patient care, or from the practitioner's error in understanding the procedure text.

Nurses and associates function within the limitations of licensure, state nurse practice act, and/or institutional policy.

<u>How to Use This Manual</u>

The first three procedures in this manual, Flexible Bronchoscopy, Flexible Bronchoscopy (Pediatric) and Rigid Bronchoscopy, are considered to be "key" procedures. Most of the other procedures in the text are based on or performed in conjunction with one of these procedures. Each key procedure is presented in detail in all aspects. The procedures that follow contain only those elements that differ from the key procedure to which each is related. For example, if the contraindications are the same as in the key procedure, they are not listed again, but the reader is referred to the key procedure for the detail. If there are contraindications in <u>addition</u> to the key procedure, those are listed.

Presenting the procedures in this manner helps to logically organize the material and prevent repetition of common information. It can also assist the staff member new to pulmonary endoscopy to readily identify those basic (key) procedures with which he/she should become familiar, and reinforces the relationships among them.

Throughout the manual, special age-specific considerations are highlighted in italics.

Procedures are categorized as primarily Diagnostic, Therapeutic or Specimen Collection, although some have aspects of more than one category. Because of its overall importance, Safety measures are outlined in section four. Section five lists the Standard Equipment required as part of the basic complement for an endoscopy setting in which pulmonary procedures are performed.

The Appendices gather supplemental material useful as a quick reference – a summary of medications commonly used in pulmonary procedures, special considerations for procedures when the patient is on mechanical ventilation and a brief overview of oxygen delivery devices. The Glossary provides definitions of pulmonary terms used in the text that may be unfamiliar to the endoscopy nurse.

Finally, the Index provides an alphabetical cross-reference to the procedures and equipment to assist you in locating specific items of interest.

Contributors and Reviewers

Education Committee Members

James Collins, BS RN CNOR - Chair
Cleveland Clinic
Cleveland, OH

Cathy S. Birn, MA RN CGRN CNOR - Co-Chair
Memorial Sloan-Kettering Cancer Center
New York City, NY

Veronica J. Besch, BSN CGRN
Saint Luke's South
Overland Park, KS

Marcia L. Bouchard, BSN RN CGRN
Southern Maine Medical Center
Biddeford, ME

Donald Cooper, MBA BSN RN CGRN LNC
Florida Hospital Heartland
Sebring, FL

Cynthia Edgelow, MSN RN CGRN
Cedars-Sinai Medical Center
Beverly Hills, CA

Darlene Gassoway, BSN RN CGRN
St. Luke's Episcopal Hospital
Houston, TX

Ingrid K. Watkins, BS RN CGRN
University of Chicago Medical Center
Chicago, IL

Joan Metze, BS BSN
Bethesda North Hospital
Cincinnati, OH

Candice Quillin, RN CGRN
St. Joseph Medical Center
Kansas City, MO

Editorial and Staff Support

Cindy M. Friis, MEd BSN RN BC
SGNA Director of Nursing Education
Chicago, Illinois

Lyndsay Graham
SGNA Education Manager
Chicago, IL

Mollie Corbett
SGNA Education Senior Associate
Chicago, IL

Part 1

DIAGNOSTIC PULMONARY PROCEDURES

Flexible Bronchoscopy (Adult)

Description

Bronchoscopy is the direct endoscopic visualization and examination of the trachea, proximal airways and segmental airways out to the third generation of branching. It allows the bronchoscopist to diagnose and treat abnormalities of the trachea and bronchial areas. It is the most common type of bronchoscopy and generally performed in a procedure room with sedation. The flexible bronchoscope consists of a flexible sheath containing cables to allow the tip to be flexed and extended, and fiberoptic fibers for transmission of images. The procedure allows the bronchoscopist to retrieve information through inspection, specimen collection or therapeutic intervention. The flexible bronchoscope may be passed transnasally, transorally or through an endotracheal or nasotracheal tube, tracheostomy or stoma.

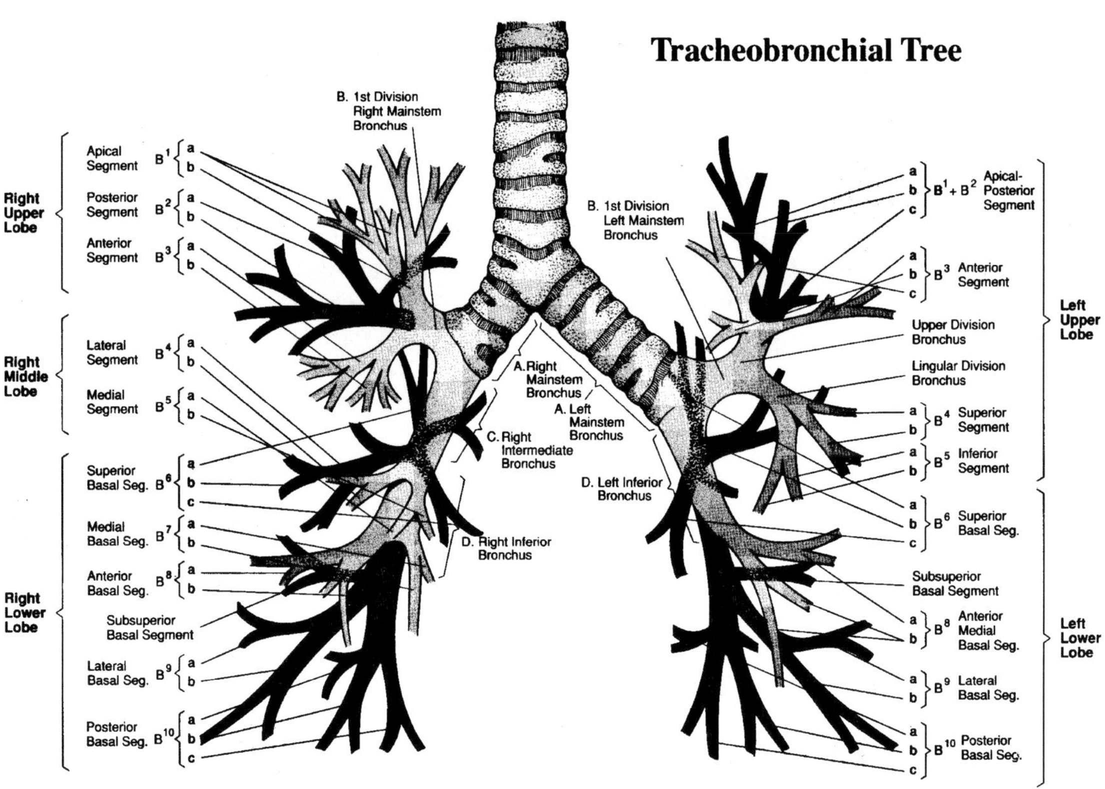

Figure 1: Tracheobronchial tree [Illustration courtesy of Boston Scientific Microvasive]

Indications

1. Abnormal radiographic study
2. Neoplastic lesions
3. Hemoptysis
4. Persistent or unexplained cough
5. Localized wheezing
6. Unresolved pneumonia
7. Lung abscess/lesion
8. Abnormal sputum cytology
9. Pulmonary infiltrate secondary to infectious etiology

10. Possible airway rupture
11. Assessment of airway status (e.g. tracheal stenosis)
12. Surveillance for lung transplant patient
13. Removal of retained or impacted secretions associated with atelectasis, pneumonia, abscess or cancer
14. Removal of foreign bodies
15. Lung lavage to improve function in patients with alveolar proteinosis
16. Insertion of endotracheal tube
17. Evaluate position of the endotracheal tube
18. Insertion of percutaneous tracheostomy tube
19. Mucosal debridement in burn patient
20. Tumor ablation, de-bulking
21. Hemostasis
22. Treatment of strictures
23. Balloon dilatation and stenting
24. Photodynamic therapy
25. Cryotherapy
26. Brachytherapy catheters
27. Bronchial Thermoplasty

Contraindications

Contraindications describe circumstances in which a particular procedure is not usually performed. In some circumstances, however, the needs of the patient may require that a procedure proceed despite the presence of the condition. The physician makes these decisions.

1. Acute asthmatic episode (active bronchospasm)
2. Current or recent myocardial infarction (MI) or hemodynamically unstable
3. Hypoxia, unless patient is intubated
4. Respiratory failure requiring high FIO_2 or PEEP
5. Bleeding diathesis – severe thrombocytopenia or coagulopathy
6. Uncooperative patient
7. Patient not NPO for 6 hours
8. Absence of informed consent

Pre-Procedure Assessment and Care

1. Confirm patient identity using two identifiers.
2. Confirm procedure to be performed, including special requests for equipment and sedation.
3. Verify informed consent for procedure and sedation/anesthesia.
4. Perform patient education of procedure and discharge instructions.
5. Verify that the outpatient has a companion or driver to assist him/her home.
6. Obtain baseline temperature, heart rate, respirations, blood pressure, oxygen saturation, capnography (facility specific) and pain level.
7. Confirm patient's medical history has been updated including allergies, current medications (anticoagulants, aspirin, NSAIDs or herbal medications) and any information pertinent to complaint.
8. Assess psychosocial factors which may affect the patient's experience during or after the procedure, e.g., home situation, language or cultural factors, past history of physical abuse.
9. Determine if the patient will need further interventions with lab studies (PT/INR, PTT) and contact the physician or follow institutional policy.
10. Verify that the patient has been NPO for a minimum of 6 hours.
11. Ensure patent venous access.
12. Administer supplemental oxygen if ordered.

13. Ascertain from patient which naris appears to be more open.
14. Administer medications as ordered.
15. Have patient's chest X-ray and/or CT films available. Communicate among team members regarding required equipment and ensure availability.
16. Administer supplemental oxygen if ordered.
17. Administer medications as ordered.

Patient Teaching

1. Determine the patient's readiness to learn and level of knowledge.
2. Explain the purpose of the procedure, the positioning, relaxation methods, techniques to be used, estimated length of the procedure and sensations the patient is likely to experience during and after the exam.
3. Instruct the patient on use of nonverbal communication, i.e., hand signals, during procedure.
4. Reassure the patient that the bronchoscope will not interfere with breathing.
5. Explain the purpose of all the equipment that is used.
6. Explain the need and rationale for the supplemental administration of oxygen during the exam.
7. Explain the effects of and rationale for the medications used and their methods of administration.
8. Review discharge instruction with patient/family prior to sedation and at discharge.
9. Document teaching and patient's understanding.

Equipment/Supplies

1. Flexible bronchoscope
2. Light source, video imaging system
3. Two suction sources
4. Monitoring system which includes blood pressure, oxygen levels, capnography (facility specfic) and cardiac rhythms
5. Oxygen and delivery device (e.g., cannula, catheter, face mask)
6. Topical anesthetic agents
7. Medications to administer per physician discretion
8. Intravenous supplies
9. Emergency airway equipment
10. Emergency medication box
11. Fluoroscopy (if ordered/indicated), lead aprons, dosimeters (refer to Safety, page 87)

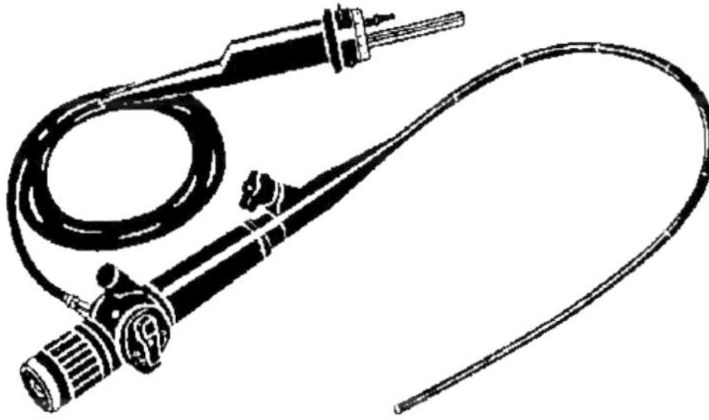

Figure 2: flexible bronchoscope

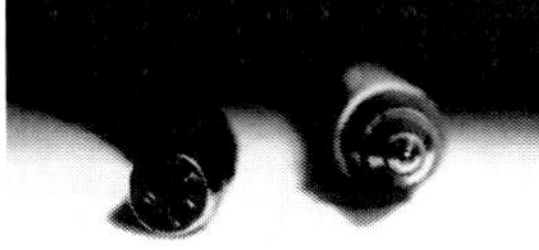

Figure 3: Bronchoscope diameter (L) compared to ball-point pen (R) [Photograph by Sharon Lesser]

Accessory Supplies

1. Biopsy forceps
2. Cytology brushes

3. Microbiology brushes
4. Aspiration needles
5. Glass slides
6. Sterile specimen containers
7. Sterile non-bacteriostatic saline
8. Slip tip syringes
9. Cytology/pathology containers with preservative
10. Labels and laboratory specimen slips
11. Suction traps, small and large (for lavage)
12. Specialized equipment for specific procedure (e.g., stenting, photodynamic therapy, bronchial thermoplasty)

Responsibilities During Procedure

1. Anesthetize upper airway as ordered (e.g., nebulizer treatment).
2. Position patient in supine position on stretcher. If fluoroscopy is needed, ensure patient is secure on fluoro table with straps as needed and protected for fluoroscopy exposure.
3. Administer oxygen with nasal cannula or facemask at liter flow per institutional policy/physician order.
4. Administer medication as directed by the physician and as permitted by state licensure and institutional policy.
5. Assist physician during procedure.
6. Monitor vital signs, capnography (if required) and oxygen saturation.
7. Assess color, warmth and dryness of skin.
8. Assess level of consciousness/mental status.
9. Assess level of comfort/response.
10. Provide emotional support to the patient.
11. Manage oral secretions.
12. Assist physician with fluoroscopy as needed.

Potential Complications

1. Hemorrhage
2. Pneumothorax
3. Hypoxemia
4. Bronchospasm
5. Cardiac dysrhythmias
6. Respiratory and/or cardiac arrest
7. Laryngospasm
8. Hypoventilation
9. Fever/infection
10. Methemoglobinemia
11. Altered hemodynamics
12. Laryngeal edema and/or injury

Post-Procedure Assessment/Care

1. Monitor vital signs (heart rate, respirations, blood pressure) and oxygen saturation.
2. Observe patient for
   a. hemorrhage
   b. change in vital signs
   c. respiratory distress
   d. chest pain or shoulder pain
   e. temperature elevation

   f. level of consciousness/mental status
   g. unexplained cyanosis
3. Maintain NPO status until gag reflex returns (approximately 1 hour after completion of the procedure).
4. Remove venous access device prior to outpatient's discharge, if applicable.
5. Provide outpatient with written discharge instructions.
6. Chest X-ray may be requested. Confirm that any X-ray ordered has been reviewed by physician prior to patient discharge.
7. Discharge outpatients who have received sedation to a person responsible for his/her transportation.

References

American Society of Gastrointestinal Endoscopy (2011). Elements to Consider when Developing a Safe Surgery Checklist for GI Ambulatory Surgical Center.

Feinsilver, S. H., & Fein, A. M. (Eds.). (1995). *Textbook of bronchoscopy.* Baltimore: Williams & Wilkins.

Gonzalez-aller de Solis, H. (1995, June). Acute methemoglobinemia: A nursing perspective. *Critical Care Nurse*, 15(3), 33-38.

Islam, Shaheen. (2011). Flexible Bronchoscopy: Equipment, procedure, and complication. P.N. Mahur & K. Wilson (Eds.), *Up To Date [On-Line].* Retrieved on Jan. 27, 2012 at http://www.uptodate.com/contents/flexible-bronchoscopy-equipment-procedure-and complication.

Maher, P. (1998). Methemoglobinemia: An unusual complication of topical anesthesia. *Gastroenterology Nursing,* 21, 173-175.

Mason, R., Broaddus, V., Murray, J., & Nadel, J. (Eds). (2005). *Textbook of Respiratory Medicine* (4th ed.), (vol. 1). Philadelphia: W.B. Saunders.

Prakash, U. B. (1994). *Bronchoscopy*. New York: Raven Press.

Sheski, F. D., & Mathur, P. N. (2001). Endoscopic options in the management of airway obstruction. In R. B. George & G. B. Epler (Eds.), *Pulmonary and critical care update on-line, 14* (lesson 21) [On-line]. Retrieved on Jan. 27, 2012 at http://www.chestnet.org/education/pccu/vol14/lesson21-22.index.html.

Wang, K., & Mehta, A. C. (2003). *Flexible bronchoscopy* (2nd ed.). Cambridge, MA: Blackwell Science.

Wilson, K. C. (2011). Flexible bronchoscopy: Indications and contraindications. P.N. Mahur & H. Hollingsworth (Eds.), *Up To Date [On-Line].* Retrieved on Jan. 27, 2012 at http://www.uptodate.com/contents/flexible-bronchoscopy-indications-and-contraindications.

Flexible Bronchoscopy (Pediatric)

Description

Flexible bronchoscopy is performed in the pediatric population for diagnostic and therapeutic purposes. Flexible bronchoscopy complements rigid or open tube bronchoscopy in the pediatric population.

Indications

1. Stridor or noisy breathing
2. Unexplained cough or wheeze
3. Hemoptysis
4. Unresolved pneumonia
5. Evaluation of endotracheal or tracheostomy tubes
6. Abnormal cry or hoarseness
7. Airway injury (trauma, thermal or toxic inhalation, toxic aspiration)
8. Removal of foreign bodies
9. Persistent or recurrent atelectasis
10. Abnormal sputum cytology
11. Recurrent or persistent pulmonary infiltrates
12. Therapeutic bronchoalveolar lavage
13. Diagnostic bronchoalveolar lavage
14. Assist in difficult intubations (cervical spine injuries, maxillofacial anomalies, facial trauma)
15. Abnormal radiographic study
16. Evaluation for bronchiolitis obliterans by biopsy

Contraindications

Contraindications describe circumstances in which a particular procedure is not usually performed. In some circumstances, however, the needs of the patient may require that a procedure proceed despite the presence of the condition. The physician makes these decisions.

1. Acute asthmatic episode (active bronchospasm)
2. Child who is uncooperative and/or cannot be sedated (general anesthesia may be indicated)
3. Coagulopathy or bleeding diathesis (relative contraindication unless biopsy is needed)
4. Severe airway obstruction or high suspicion of foreign body
5. Severe refractory hypoxemia
6. Hemodynamic instability
7. Patient not NPO for required time frame
8. Absence of informed consent of parent/guardian

Pre-Procedure Assessment/Care

1. Confirm patient identity using two identifiers.
2. Verify informed consent for procedure and sedation/anesthesia from parent or guardian.
3. Document baseline physical assessment and vital signs, including pain level, capnography if required and pulse oximetry reading.
4. Verify that the outpatient has family or legal guardian to accompany patient home.
5. Perform patient and family education of procedure and discharge instructions.
6. Obtain and document weight in kilograms. It is advisable to have available at the bedside an "Arrest Card" containing a list of appropriate doses of resuscitation medications, based on weight in kilograms.
7. Have patient's chest X-ray and/or CT films available.

8. Communicate among team members regarding required equipment and ensure availability.
9. Confirm patient's medical history has been updated including allergies, current medications (anticoagulants, aspirin, NSAIDs or herbal medications) and any information pertinent to complaint.
10. Assess psychosocial factors which may affect the patient's experience during or after the procedure, e.g., home situation, language or cultural factors, past history of physical abuse.
11. Determine if the patient will need further interventions with lab studies (PT/INR, PTT) and contact the physician or follow institutional policy.
12. Verify that the patient has been NPO for a required timeframe.
13. Place peripheral IV for sedation and emergency medication access. Assess patency of intravenous line.
14. Administer supplemental oxygen if ordered.
15. Administer medications as ordered.
16. When appropriate, immobilize the patient in order to provide security for the small child and facilitate control of the upper body.

Patient Teaching

1. Determine the patient and family's readiness to learn and level of knowledge.
2. Explain the purpose of the procedure, the positioning, relaxation methods, techniques to be used, estimated length of the procedure and sensations the patient is likely to experience during and after the exam.
3. Explain the administration of sedation to parent and child if anesthesiology not involved.
4. Using terminology appropriate to the child's developmental level, explain the procedure to the child.
5. Instruct the patient on use of nonverbal communication, i.e., hand signals, during procedure.
6. Reassure the patient/family that the bronchoscope will not interfere with breathing.
7. Explain the purpose of all the equipment that is used.
8. Explain the need and rationale for the supplemental administration of oxygen during the exam.
9. Review discharge instruction with patient/family prior to sedation and at discharge.
10. Document teaching and patient/family's understanding.

Equipment/Supplies

1. Flexible Bronchoscope of appropriate size
2. Topical anesthetic agents
3. Two suction sources
4. Medications to administer per physician discretion
5. Oxygen delivery system
6. Intravenous supplies
7. Light source, video imaging system
8. Pediatric resuscitation equipment and medications
9. Appropriately sized monitoring system which includes blood pressure, oxygen levels, capnography (facility specific) and cardiac rhythms
10. Fluoroscopy (if ordered/indicated), lead aprons, dosimeters (refer to Safety, page 87)

Accessory Supplies

1. Biopsy forceps
2. Cytology brushes
3. Microbiology brushes
4. Aspiration needles
5. Glass slides

6. Sterile specimen containers
7. Sterile non-bacteriostatic saline
8. Slip tip syringes
9. Cytology/pathology containers with preservative
10. Labels and laboratory specimen slips
11. Suction traps, small and large (for lavage)
12. Specialized equipment for specific procedure

Responsibilities During Procedure

Observe for inspiratory stridor, which can be caused by obstruction of the trachea by the bronchoscope. Maintain proper head position throughout the procedure. Decreased oxygen saturation may be secondary to improper head position, or due to side-effects of sedative medications. In the event of persistent decreased oxygen saturation, reassess the position of the head, assess for abdominal distention and consider aborting the procedure until the cause of respiratory compromise is identified and treated.

1. Continuous monitoring of vital signs, level of consciousness, capnography if required, respiratory effort and cardiac rhythm. Notify physician of any changes.
2. Anesthetize upper airway as ordered (e.g., nebulizer treatment).
3. Position patient in supine position on stretcher. If fluoroscopy is needed, ensure patient is secure on fluoro table with straps as needed and protected for fluoroscopy exposure.
4. Provide sedation per physician orders and according to institutional policy and procedure regarding sedation and analgesia.
5. Administer oxygen with nasal cannula or facemask at liter flow per institutional policy/physician order.
6. Assess color, warmth and dryness of skin.
7. Maintain position of child's head and neck.
8. Assess level of consciousness/mental status.
9. Assess level of comfort/response.
10. Provide emotional support to the patient.
11. Manage oral secretions.
12. Lightly-sedated patients may require physical restraint during the procedure to help protect the airways against damage that could occur with uncontrolled movement.

Potential Complications

1. Fever
2. Pneumothorax
3. Laryngospasm, bronchospasm
4. Transient bradycardia
5. Epistaxis
6. Hypoxemia
7. Airway or vascular trauma
8. Adverse or allergic reactions to sedation
9. Hypoventilation or apnea
10. Discomfort secondary to under-sedation
11. Hemorrhage
12. Pulmonary infiltrates
13. Cardiopulmonary arrest
14. Methemoglobinemia
15. Laryngeal edema and/or injury

Post-Procedure Assessment/Care

1. Monitor vital signs (heart rate, respirations, blood pressure) and oxygen saturation if patient received sedation and analgesia every 15 minutes x4 or until at pre-procedure levels.
2. Assess nose and oropharynx for any signs of bleeding.
3. Observe patient for
   a. respiratory distress
   b. chest pain or shoulder pain
   c. temperature elevation
   d. level of consciousness/mental status
   e. unexplained cyanosis
4. Provide parents with verbal and written post-procedure instructions, including management of fever, which is not uncommon after bronchoalveolar lavage.
5. Maintain NPO status until gag reflex returns (approximately 1 hour after completion of the procedure).
6. Observe for unexplained cyanosis.
7. Carefully monitor for return to baseline vital signs and level of consciousness. Small children and children with neurologic disability are at high risk for airway obstruction when sedated. Maintain proper head position to ensure airway patency throughout the post-procedure period.
8. Remove venous access device prior to outpatient's discharge, if applicable.
9. Provide family with written discharge instructions.
10. Chest X-ray may be requested. Confirm that any X-ray ordered has been reviewed by physician prior to patient discharge.
11. Discharge outpatients who have received sedation to a person responsible for his/her transportation.

References

American Society of Gastrointestinal Endoscopy (2011). Elements to Consider when Developing a Safe Surgery Checklist for GI Ambulatory Surgical Center.

Feinsilver, S. H., & Fein, A. M. (Eds.). (1995). *Textbook of bronchoscopy*. Baltimore: Williams & Wilkins.

Haskell, G. & Gausche-Hill, M. (2006). *PALS (Pediatric Advanced Life Support) Review*. New York: McGrawHill.

Holinger, L., Lusk, R. & Green, C. (Eds.). (1997). *Pediatric laryngology and bronchoesophagalogy*. Philadelphia: Lippincott, Williams & Wilkins.

Nicolai, T. (2001). Pediatric bronchoscopy. *Pediatric Pulmonary,* 31, 150-164.

Nussbaum, E. (2002). Pediatric fiberoptic bronchoscopy: Clinical experience with 2,836 bronchoscopies. *Pediatric Crit Care Med,* 3(2), 171-176.

Wang, K., & Mehta, A. C. (2003). *Flexible bronchoscopy* (2nd ed.).Cambridge, MA: Blackwell Science.

Rigid Bronchoscopy

Description

Rigid Bronchoscopy visualizes the trachea and proximal bronchi. It is most commonly used to manage obstructions or for interventional procedures such as insertion of airway stents. The rigid bronchoscope is a long, straight metal tube with a light at the tip. This allows direct visualization and better optics for viewing with a large suction channel which facilitates suctioning and removal of debris. It is also known as an "open tube" or "ventilating instrument." The rigid bronchscope's external diameter ranges from 2-14 millimeters and length varies from very short for pediatric patients to extra-long for adults. The distal end of the bronchoscope is beveled at an angle to assist the endoscopist in passing the instrument through the larynx. Rigid bronchoscopes are generally stainless steel tubes inserted transorally under general anesthesia.

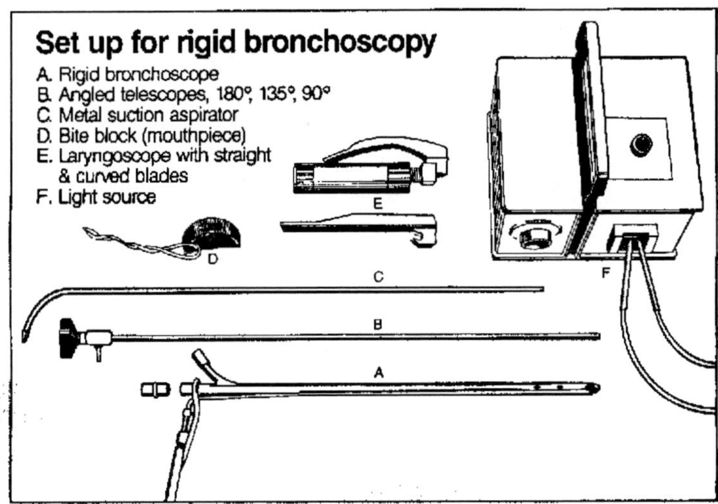

Figure 4: Setup for rigid bronchoscopy

Indications

1. Massive hemoptysis
2. Abnormal radiographic study
3. Removal of exceptionally thick, copious material or broncholiths
4. Assessment of airway involvement in burn patient
5. Strictures and stenoses of the large airways
6. Central airway obstruction
7. Biopsy of vascular tumors or bronchial adenomas
8. Endobronchial resections
9. Treatment of choice in foreign body removal in infants and small children
10. Central airway foreign body removal in adults
11. Tumor de-bulking, ablation
12. Control of hemorrhage

Contraindications

Contraindications describe circumstances in which a particular procedure is not usually performed. In some circumstances, however, the needs of the patient may require that a procedure proceed despite the presence of the condition. The physician makes these decisions.

1. Disease or trauma involving skull, jaw or cervical spine

2. NPO status less than 6 hours
3. Acute asthmatic episode (active bronchospasm)
4. Current or recent myocardial infarction (MI) or hemodynamically unstable
5. Hypoxia, unless patient is intubated
6. Respiratory failure requiring high FIO_2 or PEEP
7. Bleeding diathesis – severe thrombocytopenia or coagulopathy
8. Uncooperative patient
9. Absence of informed consent

Pre-Procedure Assessment and Care

1. Confirm patient identity using two identifiers.
2. Verify informed consent for procedure and sedation/anesthesia.
3. Confirm procedure, including special requests for equipment.
4. Perform patient education of procedure and discharge instructions.
5. Verify that sedated outpatient has a person responsible for his/her transportation.
6. Obtain baseline temperature, heart rate, respirations, blood pressure, capnography (facility specific) and oxygen saturation.
7. Confirm patient's medical history including allergies, current medications, history of head or neck trauma and information pertinent to current complaint.
8. Assess psychosocial factors which may affect the patient's experience during or after the procedure, e.g., home situation, language or cultural factors, past history of physical abuse.
9. Obtain necessary laboratory results as per institution policy and physician order. Notify physician if results are abnormal.
10. Notify physician if patient is currently on anticoagulation therapy, aspirin or non-steroidal anti-inflammatory drugs, and if laboratory results are abnormal. Determine if the patient has taken herbal preparations that affect coagulation within the last one week prior to the procedure date.
11. Verify length of NPO status (6-8 hours).
12. Establish patent intravenous access.
13. Communicate among team members regarding required equipment and ensure availability.
14. Remove dentures, if applicable.
15. Administer medications as ordered.
16. Administer supplemental oxygen as ordered.
17. Have patient's chest X-ray and/or CT films available.

Patient Teaching

1. Determine the patient's readiness to learn and level of knowledge.
2. Explain the purpose of the procedure, positioning, relaxation methods, techniques to be used, estimated length of the procedure and sensations the patient is likely to experience during and after the exam.
3. Explain the need and rationale for the use of automatic monitoring devices during the exam.
4. Explain the effects of and rationale for the use of medications and their methods of administration.
5. Explain the need and rationale for the supplemental administration of oxygen during the exam.
6. Explain the type of anesthesia (general or sedation and analgesia) to be used.

Equipment/Supplies

1. Rigid open-tube bronchoscope
2. Bronchoscope telescope with angles 180, 135, 90 degrees
3. Metal aspiration tube

4. Bite block
5. Laryngoscope with straight and curved blades
6. Light sources for bronchoscope and laryngoscope
7. Two suction sources
8. Monitoring system which includes blood pressure, oxygen levels, capnography (facility specific) and cardiac rhythms
9. Topical anesthetic agents
10. Medications to administer per physician discretion
11. Intravenous supplies
12. Oxygen with adapter for rigid scope
13. Emergency airway equipment
14. Emergency medication box

Accessory Supplies

1. Biopsy forceps including optical forceps for upper lobe biopsy
2. Cytology brushes
3. Microbiology brushes
4. Glass slides
5. Sterile specimen containers
6. Non-bacteriostatic saline
7. Slip tip syringes
8. Cytology/pathology containers with preservative
9. Laboratory specimen slips and labels
10. Suction traps, small and large (for lavage)

Responsibilities During Procedure

1. Assist with elective intubation if needed.
2. Anesthetize upper airway as ordered if using local anesthesia (nebulizer treatment, atomizer spray).
3. Administer oxygen with nasal cannula, facemask or adapter to rigid bronchoscope at liter flow per institutional policy/physician order.
4. Assist physician with medication administration if using IV sedation.
5. Position patient in proper position - supine with neck hyperextended for rigid scope. Ensure careful inspection of teeth and gums and protection of teeth with plastic mouth guard, gauze or foam rubber pads.
6. Careful attention should be noted for patients with cervical spine disease.
7. Assist physician during procedure.
8. Monitor vital signs, color, warmth and dryness of skin, level of consciousness and character of respirations. Follow institutional policy if automatic monitoring devices are used.
9. Provide emotional support if the patient is not under general anesthesia.
10. Maintain airway and manage oral secretions.
11. Assist physician with fluoroscopy as needed.
12. Properly handle, preserve and label all specimens obtained.

Potential Complications

1. Trauma to the airway resulting in bleeding, infection or perforation
2. Tracheal or esophageal perforation
3. Mouth and dental trauma
4. Pneumothorax
5. Bronchospasm or laryngospasm
6. Cardiac dysrhythmias

7. Hypoxemia
8. Laryngeal edema
9. Respiratory and/or cardiac arrest
10. Altered hemodynamics
11. Adverse effects from medications given pre- and intra-procedure

Post-Procedure Assessment/Care

1. Monitor vital signs (heart rate, respirations, blood pressure) and oxygen saturation.
2. Observe patient for
   a. hemorrhage
   b. change in vital signs
   c. respiratory distress
   d. chest pain or shoulder pain
   e. temperature elevation
   f. level of consciousness/mental status
   g. unexplained cyanosis
3. Maintain NPO status until gag reflex returns and topical anesthetic has completely worn off.
4. If the patient has received general anesthesia, observe for the return of consciousness, character of respirations, movement of extremities, color and vital signs.
5. Provide outpatient with written discharge instructions.
6. Remove venous access device prior to outpatient's discharge, if applicable.
7. Chest X-ray may be requested. Confirm that any X-ray ordered has been reviewed by physician prior to patient discharge.
8. Discharge outpatients who have received sedation to a person responsible for his/her transportation.

References

American Society of Gastrointestinal Endoscopy (2011). Elements to Consider when Developing a Safe Surgery Checklist for GI Ambulatory Surgical Center.

Beamis, J. (1999). Rigid bronchoscopy. In J. F. Beamis & P. N. Mathur (Eds.), *Interventional pulmonology*. New York: McGraw-Hill.

Colt, Henri G. 2010. Rigid Bronchoscopy. Intubation techniques. P N Mathur & K. C. Wilson (Eds.), *Up To Date,* Available: http://www.uptodate.com/contents/rigid-bronchoscopy-intubation-techniques.

Colt, Henri G. 2011. Rigid Bronchoscopy. Instrumentation. P N Mathur & K. C. Wilson (Eds.), *Up To Date,* Available: http://www.uptodate.com/contents/rigid-bronchoscopy-instrumentation

Feinsilver, S. H., & Fein, A. M. (Eds.) (1995). *Textbook of bronchoscopy*. Baltimore: Williams & Wilkins.

Ginsberg, R. J. (1995). Rigid bronchoscopy. In S. H. Feinsilver & A. .M. Fein (Eds.),*Textbook of bronchoscopy*. Baltimore: Williams & Wilkins.

Mason, R., Broaddus, V., Murray, J., & Nadel, J. (Eds). (2005). *Textbook of Respiratory Medicine* (4th ed.), (vol. 1). Philadelphia: W.B. Saunders.

Nicolai, T. (2001). Pediatric bronchoscopy. *Pediatric Pulmonary,* 31, 150-164.

Perrin, G., Colt, H. G., & Martin C. (1992). Safety of interventional rigid bronchoscopy using intravenous assisted ventilation. *Chest,* 102, 1526-1530.

Prakash, T. B. S., & Diaz-Jiminez, J. P. (1994). Rigid bronchoscopy. In U. B. S. Prakash (Ed.), *Bronchoscopy*. New York: Raven Press.

Tedder, M. & Ungerleider, R. M. (1997). Bronchoscopy. In D. C. Sabiston, Jr. & H. K. Lyerly (Eds.),*Textbook of surgery: The biological basis of modern surgical practice* (15th ed.). Philadelphia: W. B. Saunders.

Turner, J. F., Ernst, A., & Becker, H. D. (2000). Rigid bronchoscopy. *Journal of Bronchology, 7*, 171-176.

Wang, K., & Mehta, A. C. (2003). *Flexible bronchoscopy* (2nd ed.). Cambridge, MA: Blackwell Science.

Thoracentesis

Description

In thoracentesis, a needle is inserted through the intercostal space of the chest wall and into the pleural space to remove pleural fluid.

Indications

1. Relief of dyspnea secondary to large pleural effusion – most common indication
2. Sample collection for suspected malignancy/infection or other diagnostic working.

Contraindications

Contraindications describe circumstances in which a particular procedure is not usually performed. In some circumstances, however, the needs of the patient may require that a procedure proceed despite the presence of the condition. The physician makes these decisions.

Relative contraindications include the following:

1. Cardiac or hemodynamic instability
2. Respiratory insufficiency or instability (unless therapeutic thoracentesis is being performed to improve respiratory status)
3. Abnormal clotting studies
4. Uncooperative patient
5. Very small volume of fluid
6. Patient anatomy that hinders the physician from clearly identifying the appropriate landmarks
7. Chest wall cellulitis at site of puncture
8. Only one functioning lung

Pre-Procedure Assessment/Care

1. Verify informed consent.
2. Obtain baseline temperature, heart rate, respirations, blood pressure, oxygen saturation, pain level and level of consciousness.
3. Obtain patient's medical history including allergies, current medications or herbal preparations and information pertinent to current complaint.
4. Obtain necessary laboratory results (e.g., platelet count, PT, PTT, INR).
5. Administer medications as ordered.
6. Radiology findings if needed.

Patient Teaching

1. Determine the patient's readiness to learn and level of knowledge.
2. Explain the purpose of the procedure, positioning, relaxation methods, techniques to be used, estimated duration of the procedure and sensations the patient is likely to experience during and after the procedure.
3. Instruct the patient of the importance of trying not to cough during aspiration of the pleural fluid.
4. Have patient demonstrate deep breathing techniques prior to the procedure.
5. Document teaching and patient's understanding.

Equipment

1. Thoracentesis tray
2. Sterile gloves

3. Topical anesthetic
4. Sterile drapes
5. Kelly clamps
6. Stopcocks
7. Sterile specimen containers – vacuum bottles
8. Prepping solution (betadine, 2% chlorhexidine gluconate, etc.)
9. Sterile syringes
10. Lab requisition and labels
11. Heimlich valve
12. Chest tube tray and closed drainage system

Responsibilities During Procedure

1. Ensure proper time out using dual identifiers. Verify correct side of thoracentesis and verify consent.
2. Assist patient with sitting with arms resting on a pillow on an overbed table or lying partially on side (see figures below).
3. Assist physician during procedure as needed.
4. Monitor temperature, heart rate, respirations, blood pressure, oxygen saturation and pain level.
5. Observe patient for the following:
   a. change in respiratory status
   b. vasovagal response
   c. bleeding
   d. chest pain
6. Administer supplemental oxygen as ordered.
7. Provide emotional support to patient.
8. Apply a small sterile dressing to site.
9. Properly handle and label all specimens.

To prepare the patient for thoracentesis, place him in one of the three positions shown below: (1) sitting on the edge of the bed with arms on overbed table; (2) sitting up in bed with arms on overbed table; (3) lying partially on the side, partially on the back with arms over the head. These positions serve to widen the intercostal spaces and permit easy access to the pleural cavity. Using pillows as shown will make the patient more comfortable.

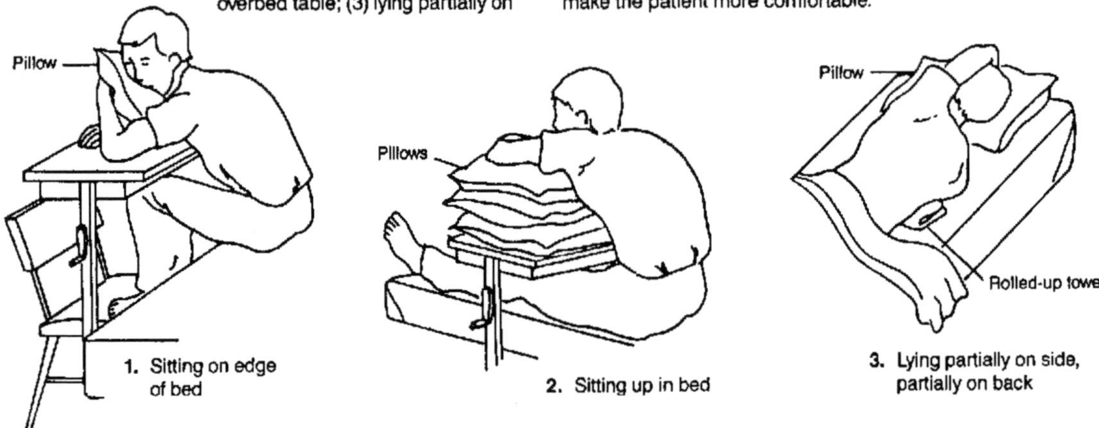

Figure 5: Positioning the patient for thoracentesis

Potential Complications

1. Pneumothorax
2. Hypovolemia
3. Vasovagal reaction
4. Pulmonary edema resulting from the rapid re-expansion of the lung

5. Air embolism
6. Hemothorax
7. Subcutaneous emphysema
8. Mediastinal shift secondary to rapid loss of fluid
9. Dyspnea
10. Spleen and liver puncture
11. Infection

Post Procedure Assessment/Care

1. Monitor vital signs and document.
2. Observe patient for signs of the following:
   a. hemorrhage
   b. change in vital signs
   c. respiratory distress
   d. chest pain
3. Check site for leakage of fluid and notify physician if necessary.
4. Document amount, character, color of fluid removed. Estimate blood loss.
5. Order tests requested by physician if applicable.
6. Chest X-ray may be requested. Confirm that any X-ray ordered has been reviewed by physician prior to patient discharge.
7. Provide outpatient with written discharge instructions.
8. Discharge patient per discharge order or discharge criteria applied.

References

Dettenmeier, P. A. (1992). *Pulmonary nursing care*. St. Louis: Mosby-Year Book.

Kozier, B., Berman, A., Erb, G. & Snyder, S. (2003). *Techniques in clinical nursing* (5th ed.). Upper Saddle River, NJ: Prentice Hall.

Krider, T., Meyer, R. (2000). *Master guide for passing the respiratory care credentialing exams* (4th ed.). Upper Saddle River, NY: Prentice-Hall.

Mason, R., Broaddus, V., Murray, J., & Nadel, J. (Eds). (2005). *Textbook of Respiratory Medicine* (4th ed.), (vol. 1). Philadelphia: W.B. Saunders.

Perel, A., & Stock, M. C. (1997). *Handbook of mechanical ventilatory support*. Baltimore: Williams & Wilkins.

Persing, G. (2000). *Advanced practitioner respiratory care review.* Philadelphia: Saunders.

Sills, J. (1995). *Respiratory care registry guide.* St. Louis: Mosby.Perry, A. G. and Potter, P. A. (2010). *Clinical Skills and Techniques* (7th ed.). St. Louis: Mosby, Inc.

Perry, A. G. and Potter, P. A. et al. (2011). *Basic Nursing* (7th ed.). St. Louis: Mosby Inc.

Smeltzer, S. and Bare, B. C. et al. (2008). *Textbook of Medical Surgical Nursing* (11th ed.). Baltimore: Lippincott, Williams, and Wilkins.

Pleural Biopsy

Description

Pleural biopsies are performed in order to evaluate a pleural effusion or for diagnostic workup. An incision or puncture with a special needle is made through the chest wall to obtain a piece of parietal pleura for analysis, culture and examination.

Indications

1. Suspected tuberculosis with unrevealing sputum studies
2. Suspected pleural based malignancy (e.g., mesothelioma)
3. Suspected primary lung malignancies

Contraindications

Contraindications describe circumstances in which a particular procedure is not usually performed. In some circumstances, however, the needs of the patient may require that a procedure proceed despite the presence of the condition. The physician makes these decisions.

1. Bleeding disorder
2. Empyema (relative) - could cause dissemination of infection

Pre-Procedure Assessment/Care

1. Same as Thoracentesis (page 17).
2. Position patient sitting or supine.
3. Clean and prep the appropriate location on the thorax in a sterile fashion.

Patient Teaching

Same as Thoracentesis (page 17).

Equipment

1. Povidone iodine, 2% chlorhexidine gluconate or whatever your facility uses
2. Injectable local anesthetic
3. #25 and #19 gauge needles for anesthesia, with 10cc syringes
4. Cope or Abrams needle (both have large outer cannula, an inner cannula that is pointed to facilitate insertion and an inner needle with a blunt end and distal hook). The Abrams needle is different only in that the needle has an additional slot on the side into which the biopsy specimen can go after it is obtained.
5. Scalpel blade (optional)
6. Thoracentesis tray
7. Specimen containers
8. Specimen preservative
9. Sterile gloves and drapes
10. Lab requisitions and labels

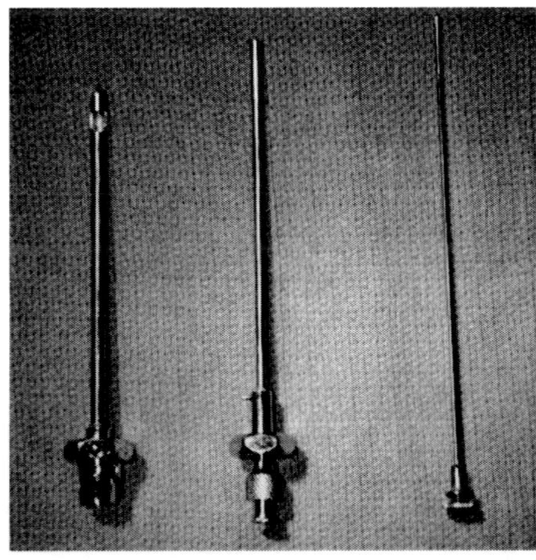

Figure 6: Abrams pleural biopsy needle [Photograph by Sharon Lesser]

Responsibilities During Procedure

Same as Thoracentesis (page 17).

Potential Complications

1. Pneumothorax
2. Hemothorax
3. Hemorrhage
4. Infection
5. Perforation of the lung
6. Mediastinal or subcutaneous emphysema

Post-Procedure Assessment/Care

1. Monitor vital signs and document procedure. Observe patient for symptoms same as Thoracentesis.
2. Chest X-ray may be requested. Confirm that any X-ray ordered has been reviewed by physician prior to patient discharge.
3. Provide outpatient with written discharge instructions.

References

Mason, R., Broaddus, V., Murray, J., & Nadel, J. (Eds). (2005). *Textbook of Respiratory Medicine* (4th ed.), (vol. 1). Philadelphia: W.B. Saunders.

McElvein, R. B. (1992). Procedures in the evaluation of chest disease. *Clinics in Chest Medicine,* 13, 1-9.

Perry, A. and Potter, P. A. (2010). *Clinical Skills and Techniques* (7th ed.). St. Louis: Mosby, Inc.

Perry, A. and Potter, P. A. et al. (2011) *Basic Nursing* (7th ed.). St. Louis: Mosby Inc.

Smelter, S. C. and Bare, B. C. et al. (2008). *Textbook of Medical Surgical Nursing* (11th ed.). Baltimore: Lippincott, Williams, and Wilkins.

Endobronchial Ultrasound

[Use in conjunction with Flexible Bronchoscopy, page 1]

Description

Ultrasound is a technology that uses high-frequency sound waves to create images of anatomical structures within the body. The sound waves are sent into the body and translated into an image by computer. Endobronchial ultrasound (EBUS) is ultrasound combined with endoscopy to obtain images in and around the bronchial tree or the lungs. EBUS allows the physician to see beyond the bronchial wall, to the diseased tissue, lymph nodes and/or lesions outside of the bronchial airways.

There are two types of EBUS which may be utilized, radial probe EBUS (R– EBUS) and convex/linear probe EBUS (C-EBUS). This is often performed with a probe passed through the biopsy channel of the bronchoscope. Technological advances now permits a Linear EBUS bronchoscope to be manufactured. This instrument permits the proceduralist to view the endoscopic image as well as the acoustic image while enabling the ability to gather tissue sampling through a variety of modalities. A radial bronchialscope is not yet available.

Indications

1. Determination of level of tumor invasion of tracheobronchial lesions for staging purposes
2. Visualization of paratracheal and peribronchial lymph nodes, and diagnosis of metastasis
3. Localization of peripheral lesions
4. Guidance of endobronchial therapy

Contraindications

Contraindications describe circumstances in which a particular procedure is not usually performed. In some circumstances, however, the needs of the patient may require that a procedure proceed despite the presence of the condition. The physician makes these decisions.

1. Same as Flexible Bronchoscopy
2. Severe pulmonary hypertension
3. Documented un-resectable disease

Pre-Procedure Assessment/Care

Same as Flexible Bronchoscopy

Patient Teaching

Same as Flexible Bronchoscopy

Equipment

1. Same as Flexible Bronchoscopy
2. Bronchoscope must have a 2.2 mm or larger working channel
3. Ultrasonography transducer probe (high-frequency with 360-degree radial viewing image)
4. Ultrasound processor

Responsibilities During Procedure

1. Same as Flexible Bronchoscopy
2. May assist physician with ultrasonic probe passage and positioning

Potential Complications

Same as Flexible Bronchoscopy

Post Procedure Assessment/Care

Same as Flexible Bronchoscopy

References

Bowling, M. R., Perry, C. D., Chin, R., Adair, N., Chatterjee, A. & Conforti, J. (2008). Endobronchial Ultrasound in the evaluation of lung cancer: A practical review and cost analysis for the practicing pulmonologist. *Southern Medical Journal.* 101(5), 534-538.

Gress, F., Savides, T., Sandler, A., Kesler, K., Conces, D., Cummings, O., Mathur, P., Ikenberry, S, Bilderback, S., & Hawes, R. (1997). Endoscopic ultrasonography: Fine-needle aspiration biopsy guided by endoscopic ultrasonography and computed tomography in the pre-operative staging of non-small cell lung cancer: A comparison study. *Annals of Internal Medicine,* 127, 604-612.

Herth,F., Becker,H.D., Lo Cicerio III, J. & Ernst, A. (2002). Endobronchial Ultrasound in Therapeutic Bronchoscopy. *Eur Respir J,* 20, 118-121.

Hurter, T., & Hanrath, P. (1992). Endobronchial sonography. *Thorax,* 47, 565-567.

Kurimoto, N., Murayama, M., Yoshioka, S., Nishisaka, T., Inai, K., & Dohi, K. (1999). Assessment of usefulness of endobronchial ultrasonography in determination of depth of tracheobronchial tumor invasion. *Chest,* 115, 1500-1506.

Orens, J. B., Daly, B., & Britt, E. J. (1997). Endobronchial ultrasound via the fiberoptic bronchoscope. *Seminars in Respiratory and Critical Care Medicine,* 18(6), 593-601.

Pierson, D. (Ed.). (1993).Fiberoptic bronchoscopy assisting [clinical practice guideline]. *Respiratory Care,* 38, 1173-1178.

Yuji, T., Kawahaia, M., Agawaia, M., Furusi, K., Yamamoto, S., Ueru, K., Hosoe, S., Atagi, S., Kawaguchi, Y., Tsuchiyama, T., Naka, N., Kiskio, K., Miki, M., & Mori, T. (2000). Ultrasound-guided flexible bronchoscopy for the diagnosis of tumor invasion to the bronchial wall and mediastinum. *Journal of Bronchology,* 7, 127-132.

Electromagnetic Navigation Bronchoscopy

[Use in conjunction with Flexible Bronchoscopy, page 1]

Description

Electromagnetic Navigation Bronchoscopy (ENB) is a specialized bronchoscopic procedure utilizing electromagnetic guidance. The foundation encompasses a real-time, image-directed localization, allowing physicians to drive/steer a bronchoscope to peripheral lung lesions. This entire process affords the physician to sample lesions for diagnosis and staging, as well as prepare them for treatment.

The ENB process begins with the patient having a digitalized CT scan of the chest to locate a deep lesion. The physician loads the CT scan study into a planning software system (unique lap top computer) that creates a 3-dimensional "roadmap" of the patient's lungs. The physician plans/plots a pathway to the lesion. Actual anatomic landmarks can be referenced as well as the targeted site. The actual plan is saved on a USB drive or CD and then plugged into the Electromagnetic System to begin the procedure. The patient is then placed on a stretcher over an electromagnetic board, with tracking triplet sensors put in place on the patient's chest. These sensors will show the position of the sensor probe. This micro sensor probe is inserted through the working channel of the bronchoscope into the airways. The true pathway, and/or landmarks are identified by the probe bronchoscopically, registered in the system and aligned with data from the CT scan. The Locatable Guide (LG) can then be directed in "real-time" to the target lesion. Once at the target lesion, the locatable guide catheter is removed, with an Extended Working Channel left in place. Specimen tools/accessories can now be placed through the extended working channel to collect tissue for testing and diagnosis. Also, the physician can place fiducial markers for future radiation treatments.

Indications

1. Assess peripheral lung lesions/nodules/aneurysms; lesion size and location beyond the scope of conventional bronchoscopy
2. Use in patients not suitable for surgery or other invasive procedures (e.g., CT-guided Trans Thoracic Node Assessment)
3. Small lesions (8mm smallest); ideal size > 2 cm
4. Staging lymph nodes (subcarinal and mediastinal)
5. Placement of radio-surgical markers for radiation treatments/therapy
6. Placement of markers for VATS (Video Assisted Thoracic Surgery)
7. Delivery of radiation sources (Brachytherapy)

Contraindications

Contraindications describe circumstances in which a particular procedure is not usually performed. In some circumstances, however, the needs of the patient may require that a procedure proceed despite the presence of the condition. The physician makes these decisions.

1. Pediatric patients
2. Patients with pacemakers, AICDs, or other electrically or magnetically activated implanted medical devices
3. Patients whose size prevents the patient sensing probes from being in the required sensing field
4. Profound anatomic variations (e.g., COPD, prior surgery)
5. Procedure may only be done by credentialed ENB physicians
6. Benefit versus risk assessed with a pregnant patient because of any radiation exposure

Pre-Procedure Assessment/Care

1. Same as for Flexible Bronchoscopy.
2. Patients should be off of any "blood thinning" medications for 7 days prior to procedure.

Patient Teaching

1. Same as for Flexible Bronchoscopy.
2. Patient may be sedated with General Anesthesia; therefore, the anesthesiologist providing sedation must explain risks and benefits of General Anesthesia. Patient may have a "sore throat" more than usual or "hoarseness" due to the ETT.
3. Explain use and placement of electromagnetic sensors on the patient's chest prior to the procedure.
4. Patient can expect to be in PACU for recovery and either sent back to original unit or a Day Surgery Unit for completion of recovery and discharge.

Equipment

Important Note: Procedure room that will be used for ENB must be "mapped" with all possible equipment that could be used placed in designated locations. This occurs so the electromagnetic field is not disrupted; you cannot just set all equipment up in an alternate room unless it has been appropriately "mapped."

1. Same as for Flexible Bronchoscopy
2. Therapeutic Bronchoscope (2.8mm working channel)
3. Fluorosopy equipment: C-Arm, image tower and lead aprons
4. Electromagnetic Navigation System Tower (i.e., i Logic/Superdimension system) with appropriate cables
5 Electromagnetic Navigation Location Board
6. Special fluoroscopy stretcher marked for placement of Location Board
7. Superdimension Kit (Electromagnetic Navigation specialty kit): includes Extended Working Channel (EWC), Locatable Guide (LG), bronchoscope adapter and clip
8. Set of Patient Sensor Triplets; paper tape
9. ENB specialized accessories: forceps, cytology brushes, needlebrushes, FNA needle, microbiology brushes
10. "White-Out" solution with permanent marker to "mark" all accessories
11. Anesthesia equipment set-up for General Anesthesia
12. 8.5fr ETT
13. ETT adapter
14. Luer lock style syringes for normal saline/cold normal saline/empty ones

Responsibilities Surrounding Procedure

An Endoscopy Technician and/or RN specialty trained for the ENB procedure will position all equipment in the room and set it up accordingly.

A. Pre-Procedure Set-up and Process:

1. Power system on/Open screen/Select procedure
2. Check room configuration to system picture, observe minimum distances (nothing metal within 2 feet of Location Board)
3. Check location board position
4. Check cable connections – video input, patient sensor triplets, locatable guide, footswitch, location board
5. Confirm therapeutic bronchoscope (2.8mm working channel)

6. Attach bronchoscope adapter and clip
7. Mark endoscopic tool length
8. Insert flash drive, load plan and enter patient data
9. Attach patient sensors to patient's chest after patient is placed on specialized fluoroscopy bed; patient's chest must be within arrow-marked lines on stretcher; confirm status view
10. RN and/or Anesthesiologist will connect patient to vital sign monitors
11. Anesthesiologist will intubate patient; RN may assist with this process

B. **Intra-Procedure Process**: (procedure will require either 1 technician/1RN or 2 RNs)
   1. Endoscopy Technician or RN will:
      a. Be immediate assistant to physician for handling scope/ENB accessories/and in specimen acquisition; depending on institution and/or physician preference, the Endoscopy Technician or RN may manipulate/control the Locatable Guide
      b. Be liaison staff member to assist with transferring specimens to second RN who processes the specimens
      c. Adjust settings on ENB computer per physician's direction
      d. Mark fluoroscopic images per physician's directions on radiologic screen
      e. Assist anesthesiologist with patient as needed
   2. RN only will:
      a. Process specimens
      b. Document procedure

C. **Safety Considerations**:
   1. Patient must not have electrical or magnetically activated implanted devices.
   2. Cannot install other software into the ENB system.
   3. Cannot change the configuration of the special procedure room, including introduction of new metallic equipment or movement of existing equipment; this can affect the accuracy of the system.
   4. No cell phones, pagers and related items can be turned on in the working field.
   5. The minimum distance between the System Tower and the Location Board is 50cm.
   6. The minimum distance between the Locatable Guide handle and the Location Board is 40cm.
   7. Before switching any ECG units included in the original mapping of the room, verify compatibility of the new ECG with the ENB system.
   8. The Locatable Guide, Extended Working Channel, Bronchoscope Clip and Adapter are all single use.
   9. The tip of the LG must protrude 5mm (+/- 3mm) from the end of the EWC.
   10. Never operate the LG without the EWC attached. Damage to any system accessories can cause tissue irritation and possible injury to the bronchial airways.
   11. Use of bronchoscopic tools that do not comply with specifications have the potential to damage the EWC and potential injury to the bronchial airways.
   12. Patient should be immobile for 5 seconds from the time the "Finish" button is clicked.
   13. Patient must be kept in a supine position and still during entire procedure, as excessive patient movement can affect the accuracy of the system and result in patient injury.
   14. CT-to-body divergence values must not be more than 10mm. Greater values can affect the accuracy of the system and cause potential patient injury.
   15. After any replacement of the LG during the procedure, repeat visual registration verification must be done.
   16. Any movement of the bronchoscope while the LG is being removed and the EWC is locked in place will affect the position of the EWC, moving it off target. The LG will need to be reinserted and a re-navigation to the target is imperative.

17. Fluoroscopy on at least 2 perpendicular angles should be used to verify the location of the LG at the target.
18. If any resuscitation equipment must be applied to the patient, switch off the main power of the ENB system, remove Patient Sensors and the LG away from the patient's body.

Potential Complications

1. Same as for Flexible Bronchoscopy.
2. Refer to Safety Considerations for ENB above.

Post-Procedure Assessment/Care

1. Same as for Flexible Bronchoscopy.
2. Assist anesthesiologist or CRNA with patient as needed in monitoring vital signs, providing supplemental oxygen, moving patient to regular stretcher for transport to PACU, accompanying anesthesia personnel to PACU with patient.

Post-Procedure Process (after patient is out of room)

1. Same as for Flexible Bronchoscopy.
2 Remove Location Board from specialized stretcher; store in safe, protected compartment on the ENB Tower.
3. Wipe down all permanent ENB Tower cables with hospital approved disinfectant and store appropriately on Tower. Do not leave cables hanging loose.

References

Edell, E. and Krier-Morrow, D. (2010). Navigational Bronchoscopy, New Current Procedural Technology Codes Effective 2010. *Chest*, 137(2), 450-454.

Feller-Kopman, D. (2011). Navigational Bronchoscopy. *Journal of Bronchology and Interventional Pulmonology*, 18(3), 209-210.

Lee, R. and Ost, D. (2010). Advanced Bronchoscopic Techniques for Diagnosis of Peripheral Pulmonary Lesions. *Interventional Pulmonary Medicine* (2nd ed.). New York: Informa Healthcare USA, Inc.

Mahajan, A.K., Patel, S., Hogarth, D.K., et al. (2011). Electromagnetic Navigational Bronchoscopy. An Effective and Safe Approach to Diagnose Peripheral Lung Lesions Unreachable by Conventional Bronchoscopy in High-Risk Patients. *Journal of Bronchology and Interventional Pulmonology*, 18(2), 133-137.

Merritt, S. A., Gibbs, J.D., Yu, K., et al. (2008) Image-Guided Bronchoscopy for Periperal Lung Lesions, A Phantom Study. *Chest*, 134(5), 1017-1025.

Morgan, R. and Ernst, A. (2009). Advanced Diagnostic Bronchoscopy. In Ernst, A. (Ed.), *Introduction to Bronchoscopy*. New York: Cambridge University Press.

Shah, P. (2012). *Atlas of Flexible Bronchoscopy*. London: Hodder Arnold.

Fluorescence Bronchoscopy

[Use in conjunction with Flexible Bronchoscopy, page 1]

Description

Fluorescence Bronchoscopy is used to identify pre-invasive lesions (metaplasia, dysplasia and carcinoma in situ) in the bronchial epithelium in the tracheobronchial tree that may not be seen under white light bronchoscopy. Abnormal bronchial tissue exhibits a weaker green/red fluorescence than normal healthy tissue when illuminated with a blue light. Tissue samples can then be taken of these questionable areas. In identifying and treating these lesions the hope is to decrease squamous cell carcinoma of the tracheobronchial tree.

Indications

1. Patients that have high grade sputum atypia but no radiological abnormalities seen
2. Surveillance of patients with previously diagnosed pre-invasive lesions
3. Patients with early invasive lung cancer who are being considered for endobronchial or surgical treatment

Contraindications

Contraindications describe circumstances in which a particular procedure is not usually performed. In some circumstances, however, the needs of the patient may require that a procedure proceed despite the presence of the condition. The physician makes these decisions.

1. Same as Flexible Bronchoscopy
2. Documented un-resectable disease

Pre-Procedure Assessment/Care

Same as Flexible Bronchoscopy

Equipment

1. Autofluorescence Imaging System

Responsibilities During Procedure

1. Same as Flexible Bronchoscopy
2. May assist the physician with the Autofluorescence Imaging System

Potential Complications

Same as Flexible Bronchoscopy

Post-Procedure Assessment/Care

Same as Flexible Bronchoscopy

References

Banerjee, A. (2010). Fluorescence Bronchoscopy. Retrieved on Feb. 3, 2012 from www.uptodate.com.

Banerjee, PH, Rabbitts, G. J. (2002). Fluorescence Bronchoscopy: Clinical Dilemmas and Research Opportunities. *Thorax*; 58, 266-271.

George, PJM. (1999). Fluorescence Bronchoscopy for the Early Detection of Lung Cancer. *Thorax*, 54, 180-183.

Kennedy, T. C., Lam, S., Hirsch, F. (2001). Review of Recent Advances in Fluorescence Bronchoscopy in Early Localization of Central Airway Lung Cancer. *The Oncologist*, 6, 257-262.

Part 2

THERAPEUTIC PULMONARY PROCEDURES

Intrabronchial Brachytherapy

[Use in conjunction with Flexible Bronchoscopy, page 1]

Description

Brachytherapy refers to the placement of a radioactive source within or in close proximity to a malignancy in order to provide local or internal radiation therapy. This approach assures the highest dose of radiation to the tumor site. In Intrabronchial Brachytherapy, a polyethylene catheter is passed transnasally under the direct visualization of bronchoscopy, to a site in close proximity to the tumor. This catheter is called an afterloading catheter. Upon completion of the bronchoscopy, radioactive seeds will be inserted through the catheter, usually by radiation oncology services.

Indications

The major use of Intrabronchial Brachytherapy is for the palliation of symptoms related to airway obstruction.

1. Inoperable/obstructive primary or metastatic endobronchial tumors
2. Secondary treatment for lung cancer as an adjunct to surgery, chemotherapy or external beam radiation therapy
3. Treatment for tumor recurrence when the surrounding tissue has not reached maximum radiation dose tolerance
4. Palliation of symptoms such as pain, pulmonary obstruction, hemoptysis, dyspnea and cough

Contraindications

Contraindications describe circumstances in which a particular procedure is not usually performed. In some circumstances, however, the needs of the patient may require that a procedure proceed despite the presence of the condition. The physician makes these decisions.

1. Same as Flexible Bronchoscopy
2. The patient has already received a total radiation tissue tolerance for the area needing the treatment

Pre-Procedure Assessment/Care

1. Same as Flexible Bronchoscopy
2. Administer medication as ordered to control cough. Coughing and bronchospasm could dislodge catheter from the area to be treated.

Patient Teaching

1. Same as Flexible Bronchoscopy
2. Education about the radiation treatment itself is the responsibility of radiation oncology personnel.

Equipment

1. Same as Flexible Bronchoscopy
2. Flexible brachytherapy catheter(s)
3. Tape

Responsibilities During Procedure

Same as Flexible Bronchoscopy

Potential Complications

1. Same as Flexible Bronchoscopy
2. Complications may occur either early or late in treatment
3. Early complications are usually related to bronchoscopy or catheter placement
4. Late complications may include radiation bronchitis and airway stenosis
5. Bronchospasm
6. Intolerance of the catheter(s)
7. Excessive radiation-induced bronchitis
8. Abcess or transesophagel fistula formation between the esophagus, pleura or bronchial system
9. Hemorrhage

Post-Procedure Assessment/Care

1. Same as Flexible Bronchoscopy
2. Mark catheter at point where it exits the nose. Tape catheter in place.

References

Dow, K. H., Bucholtz, J. D., Iwamoto, R. R., Fisler, V. K., & Hilderley, L. J. (1997). Principles of brachytherapy. In C. Dunne-Daly (Ed.), *Nursing care in radiation oncology* (2nd ed.). Philadelphia: Saunders.

Feinsilver, S., & Fein, A. M. (Eds.). (1995). *Textbook of bronchoscopy*. Baltimore: Williams & Wilkins.

Mason, R., Broaddus, V., Murray, J., & Nadel, J. (Eds). (2005). *Textbook of Respiratory Medicine* (4th ed.), (vol. 1). Philadelphia: W.B. Saunders.

Pass, H., Carbone, D., Johnson, D., Minna, J., & Turrisi, A. (2004). *Lung Cancer: Principles and Practice* (3rd ed.). Philadelphia: Lippincott, Williams & Wilkins.

Rosenzweig, KE, Movas, B., Bradley, J. et al. (2009). ACR appropriateness criteria on nonsurgical treatment for non-small cell lunch cancer: poor performance status or palliative intent. *Journal of the American College of Radiology*, 6(2), 85-95.

Sheski, F. D., & Mathur, P. N. (2001). Endoscopic options in the management of airway obstruction. In R. B. George & G. B. Epler (Eds.), *Pulmonary and critical care update on-line, 14* (lesson 21) [On-line]. Available: http://www.chestnet.org/education/pccu/vol14/lesson21-22.index.html

Wang, K., & Mehta, A. C. (2012). *Flexible bronchoscopy* (3rd ed.). Cambridge, MA: Blackwell Science.

Chest Tube Insertion (Thoracostomy)

Description

The thoracic cavity is a closed air space, and any disruption in the loss of negative pressure within the intrapleural space (air or fluid) can cause symptoms. The chest tube, placed between ribs, reestablishes normal intrapleural and intrapulmonic pressure by evacuating air (pneumothorax) or fluid (effusion, pus, blood). Chest tubes are sterile catheters and come in a varying array of sizes and diameters. Chest tubes range in size from very small (12 to 18 French) to large (as high as 42 French). The larger chest tubes are used to drain more turbid, tenacious effusions (pus, blood) or large pneumothoraces. The size of the tube placed is determined by the condition. Chest tubes also come in different configurations (curved or straight) and different materials (PVC or silicone) and are available with Heparin coating to reduce friction on insertions.

The overall goal of the chest tube is to promote lung expansion, restore adequate oxygenation and ventilation and prevent complications.

Indications

1. Pneumothorax
2. Hemothorax
3. Empyema
4. Pleural effusion
5. Chylothorax
6. Hemopneumothorax
7. Tension pneumothorax
8. Prevent or mitigate post-op complications.

Contraindications

Contraindications describe circumstances in which a particular procedure is not usually performed. In some circumstances, however, the needs of the patient may require that a procedure proceed despite the presence of the condition. The physician makes these decisions.

1. Coagulopathy (due to intrinsic disease or anti-coagulation)
2. Hepatohydrothorax

Pre-procedure Assessment/Care

1. Verify informed consent.
2. Obtain baseline vital signs (including pulse oximetry) and establish continuous vital signs monitoring.
3. Obtain patient's medical history, including allergies, current medications (including anticoagulants, aspirin, NSAIDs and herbal medications) and any information pertinent to current complaint.
4. Determine if patient will need further interventions with lab studies (PT/INR, PTT) and contact physician or follow institutional policy.
5. Confirm NPO status.
6. Establish patent venous access.
7. Provide supplemental O_2 if needed (or determine if patient needs intubation).

Patient Teaching

1. Same as Flexible Bronchoscopy.
2. Explain the need and rationale for maintenance of sterile conditions and patient's position during the procedure.
3. Explain to the patient that lung re-expansion during the procedure may cause cough.
4. Assure the patient that the initial pain of tube insertion will diminish as the lung expands.
5. Instruct patient and responsible party about activities as prescribed while maintaining the drainage system below the level of the chest.

Equipment

1. Chest tube tray may include:
   a. sterile towels and drapes
   b. injectable local anesthetic
   c. sutures with tapered or cutting needle
   d. needle holder
   e. large Kelly clamps (2)
   f. medium Kelly clamps (2)
   g. large straight suture scissors (one)
   h. basin for prep solution
   i. sterile gauze pads 4X4's
2. Properly-assembled closed chest drainage system according to manufacturer's instruction
3. Heimlich one way valve
4. Chest tube, 12 to 42 French
5. Means of securing chest tube to drainage tube (e.g., tape, elastoplast, etc.)
6. Occlusive dressing
7. Vaseline gauze
8. Suction source
9. Antiseptic solution (betadine, 2% chlorhexidine gluconate per institutional policies)
10. Skin barrier protection
11. Sterile gloves
12. Sterile water
13. "Y" connector

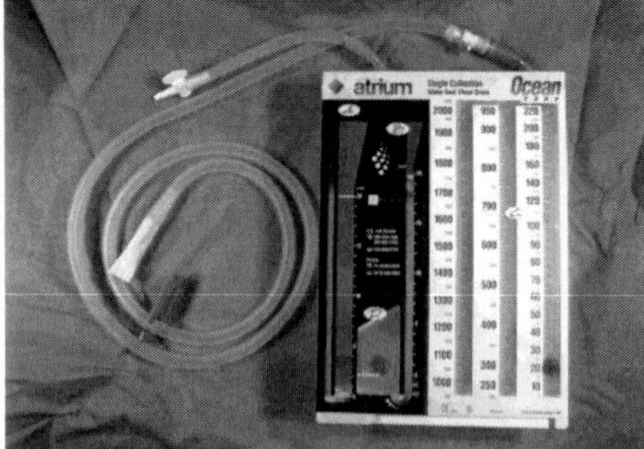

Figure 7: closed chest drainage system [Photo by David Crandall]

Responsibilities During Procedure

1. Same as Flexible Bronchoscopy.
2. Ensure proper time out using dual identifiers. Verify correct side of chest tube placement and verify consent.
3. Position patient as directed.
4. Provide patient reassurance and support, even in an emergent situation.
5. Set up chest tube drainage unit (CDU) according to manufacturer instructions.

Potential Complications

1. Hemorrhage from trauma to chest wall, visceral structures
2. Damage to lung parenchyma if tube is inserted into lung tissue and not into pleural space
3. Hypotension with removal of large effusion
4. Infection/abscess at entry site and at placement site in pleural space
5. Subcutaneous emphysema
6. Cardiac arrest from non-expanded lung/tension pneumothorax
7. Incorrect tube placement or chest tube kinking, clogging or dislodgement from chest wall

Post-Procedure Assessment/Care

1. Same as Flexible Bronchoscopy.
2. Apply occlusive dressing.
3. Ensure chest tube is securely attached to the drainage system. Tape all connections and secure tube to chest wall.
4. Observe chest tube and record initial drainage (amount, color, rate of flow).
5. Chest X-ray may be requested. Confirm that any X-ray ordered has been reviewed by physician prior to patient discharge.
6. Connect drainage system to suction, if ordered.
7. Place CDU below level of patient chest.

References

Bauman, M. and Handley, M. (2011). Chest Tube care: The more you know, the easier it gets. *American Nurses Today*, 9, 27-32.

Carroll, P. (2000). Exploring chest drain options. *RN, 63*(10), 50-59.

Durai, R., et al. (2010). Manageing a Chest Tube and Drainage System. *AORN*, 2, 275-283.

Dettenmeier, P. A. (1992). *Pulmonary nursing care*. St. Louis: Mosby.

Devanand, A. et al. (2004). Simple aspiration versus chest-tube insertion in the management of primary spontaneous pneumothorax. *Respiratory Medicine,* 98, 579-590.

Gilbert, T. B., McGrath, B. J., & Soberman, M. (1993). Chest tubes: Indications, placement, management, and complications. *Intensive Care Medicine,* 8, 73-86.

Hart, J. Chest Tube Insertion. A.D.A.M., Health on the Net Foundation. Last updated 9/19/2011. VeriMed Healthcare Network.

Hudson, K. "Chest Trauma: Nursign care and management". Retrieved on December 21, 2011 from www.Dynamic NursingEducation.com.

Perry, A. G. and Potter, P. A., et al. (2011). *Basic Nursing* (7th ed.). St. Louis: Mosby Inc.

Perry, A. and Potter, P. A. (2010). *Clinical Skills and Techniques* (7th ed.). St. Louis, Mosby, Inc.

Pruitt, B. (2008). Clearing the air with Chest Tubes. *Men in Nursing*, 12, 32-37.

Schoenenberger, R. A., Haefeli, W. E., Weiss, P., & Ritz, R. (1993). Evaluation of conventional chest tube therapy for iatrogenic pneumothorax. *Chest,* 104, 1770-1772.

Smeltzer, S., Bare, B., et al. (2008). *Textbook of Medical Surgical Nursing* (11th ed.). Baltimore: Lippincott, Williams, and Wilkins.

Cryotherapy

[Use in Conjunction with Flexible Bronchoscopy, page 1, or Rigid Bronchoscopy, page 11]

Description

Cryotherapy causes cold-induced tissue/cell destruction by repeated cycles of cold application followed by thawing. Factors affecting destruction include rates of freezing and thawing (rapid freezing and slow thawing produces maximum cell death), number of freeze-thaw cycles (repeating cycles increases the amount of destruction) and length of freezing time and thawing time. Unlike electrocautery and APC, cryotherapy effects occur mainly hours later after application (vascular effects occur 6-12 hours post application). However, the sheer contact between the cryoprobe and tissue leads to immediate adherence between surfaces. Thus, it is excellent for foreign body removal.

Indications

Curative or palliative treatment of:

1. Hemoptysis
2. Endotracheal lesions – primary or metastatic malignancy (primary candidates have tumors that are accessible via the bronchoscope with polypoid, short length, large endobronchial component, some visibility beyond the lesion and functional lung distal to the lesion, and are otherwise not candidates for curative surgical resection)
3. Removal of foreign bodies
4. Removal of mucus plugs
5. Removal of blood clots
6. Treatment of granulation tissue
7. Treatment of stenosis – alone or with other adjunctive treatment (balloon dilation, stent placement)
8. Treatment of benign airway tumors
9. Dielafoy lesions
10. Mobile broncholiths
11. Vascular Tumors (no residual stenosis)

Pre-Procedure Assessment and Care

Same as Flexible Bronchoscopy, or Rigid Bronchoscopy.

Patient Teaching

1. Same as Flexible Bronchoscopy, or Rigid Bronchoscopy.
2. Patient may experience a self-limiting fever brought on by the inflammatory response of cell death.
3. With excessive sloughing of tissue, dyspnea and coughing can result; Flexible bronchoscopy may be needed several days after the cryotherpy to assist in clearing the airways.

Equipment

1. If using the flexible fiberoptic bronchoscope, refer to Flexible Bronchoscopy (see page 1). Both a regular and therapeutic bronchoscope are essential.
2. If using the rigid bronchoscope, refer to Rigid Bronchoscopy (see page 11)
3. Retrieval instruments, i.e., biopsy forceps, grasping forceps
4. Coolant (nitrous oxide, or CO2) with console, regulator and foot pedal
5. Cryoprobes of various sizes

6. Clock with a second hand
7. Sterile water and basin

Set-up

1. Remove and save sterilizing cap from cryoprobe selected by physician.
2. Verify the presence of O-rings. Damaged O-ring can cause gas leak at cylinder.
3. Screw the neck of the cryoprobe tightly onto the console. The venting valve can be in any position.
4. Fully open the valve (turn to the left) to the coolant. The gauge should be at the appropriate level.
5. Turn the main switch on. An indicator light and a "Ready" light will be illuminated.
6. Step on foot pedal (note "Freeze" light) for 45-60 seconds. Check the freezing power and leaking by immersing the probe tip in sterile water. Note formation of ice ball.
7. Release foot pedal. Note "Defrost" light activation.
8. Some models of cryoprobes do not have a "Defrost" light. If this feature is absent, perform the following steps:
   a. Test the cryoprobe before use, timing how long it takes for the ice ball to thaw.
   b. When applying to tissue, keep the physician verbally informed of the time elapsed since the probe was deactivated.
9. During procedure, do not withdraw cryoprobe into scope for 45-60 seconds or until the ice ball has thawed. After the "Defrost" light goes off, the unit is no longer pressurized.

Responsibilities During Procedure

1. Same as Flexible Bronchoscopy.
2. Remove debris from cryoprobe tip as needed.
3. If working on an intubated patient, after tissue is blanched, the swivel adaptor is disconnected from the ETT. Then the physician will pull the scope and probe out simultaneously from the ETT. Assist in immediately replacing the swivel adaptor to the ETT, so there is minimal interruption in ventilation of the patient.

Post Procedure

1. Close the coolant tank tightly (turn to the right).
2. Step on foot pedal until pressure is totally released. Ensure the gauge reading is at appropriate level, or zero. Gas pressure must be released in order to prevent liquid formation which can damage the probe.
3. Turn off the main switch. The indicator light will go out.
4. Remove the cryoprobe from the machine and tightly replace the sterilization cap.
5. Steam autoclave the individual probe in its designated tray.

Post-Procedure Assessment/Care

Same as Flexible Bronchoscopy.

References

Greenwald, B. and Dumot, J. A. (2011). Cryotherapy for Barrett's esophagus and esophageal cancer. *Current Opinion in Gastroenterology*, 27(4), 363-367.

Jinwoo, L, Young S. P., Seok-Chung, Y. (2011). The endoscopic cryotherapy of lung and bronchila tumors: A systemic review- can we expect a new era of cryotherapy in lung cancer? *The Krean Journal of Internal Medicine*, 26(2), 132-134.

Prakash, U. (1999). Advances in bronchoscopic procedures. *Chest*, 116, 1403-1408.

Skeski, F.D., & Mathur, P.N. (1999). Flexible bronchoscopy in the 21st century, cryotherapy, electrocautery and brachytherapy. *Clinics in Chest Medicine*, 20 (1), 123-130.

Sheski, F.D., & Mathur, P.N. (2001). Endoscopic options in the management of airway obstruction. In R.B. George & G.B. Epler (Eds), *Pulmonary and critical care update on-line,* 14, (lesson 21) [On-line]. Retrieved on Jan. 17, 2012 from http://www.chestnet.org/education/pccu/vol14/lesson21-22.index.html.

Endobronchial Electrosurgery/Coagulation
(Monopoloar, Bipolar, Heater Probe, Argon Plasma Coagulation)

[Use in conjunction with Flexible Bronchoscopy, page 1, And Rigid Bronchoscopy, page 11]

Description

Electrocautery refers to a technique of tissue alteration/destruction by application of heat via an electric current.

A. Monopolar Electrosurgery: An adjunct procedure to bronchoscopy which uses high frequency current (in a contact technique) to produce three basic effects: cutting (vaporization), fulguration and desiccation (coagulation). Distinct levels of tissue response depend on power used, length of time of application, contact surface area and type of tissue treated.

B. Bipolar Coagulation: A specialized system that consists of an electrosurgical generator with a bipolar output mode and a series of probes (having active and return electrodes side-by-side at the tip) and instruments suitable for producing electrosurgical coagulation of a limited depth.

C. Argon Plasma Coagulation (APC): A non-contact monopolar electrosurgical unit that ionizes a stream of argon gas for hemostasis and tissue devitalization. APC provides a more homogeneous but superficial effect. Application is versatile with axial, radial and retrograde options.

Indications

A. Monopolar Electrosurgery:
   1. Presence of endobronchial polyps or masses
   2. Presence of bleeding
   3. Devitalization of tumor in-growth and overgrowth (e.g., in expandable metal stents) or granulation tissue after stent placement
   4. Benign airway stenosis; Subglottic stenosis
   5. Palliation of unresectable malignant tumors
   6. Possible curative treatment for carcinoma in situ
   7. Herniated tracheal rings

B. Bipolar Coagulation
   1. Active bleeding lesions in the lung

C. Argon Plasma Coagulation
   1. Hemostasis
   2. Tissue devitalization of tumors
   3. Devitalization of tumor in-growth and overgrowth (e.g., in expandable metal stents) or granulation tissue after stent placement
   4. Benign airway stenosis
   5. Airway lesions requiring sharp angle treatment
   6. Papillomatosis
   7. Post-infectious airway stenosis

Contraindications

Contraindications describe circumstances in which a particular procedure is not usually performed. In some circumstances, however, the needs of the patient may require that a procedure proceed despite the presence of the condition. The physician makes these decisions.

A. Monopolar Electrosurgery
   1. Coagulopathy

Therapeutic Pulmonary Procedures

2. Uncooperative patient
3. Extrinsic compression of airways

B. Bipolar Coagulation
1. Uncooperative patient
2. Massive hemorrhage which requires immediate surgery
3. Inadequate visualization of the bleeding site

C. Argon Plasma Coagulation
1. Uncooperative patient
2. Massive hemorrhage that requires immediate surgery
3. Inability to visualize probe tip
4. Extrinisic compression of airways

Pre-Procedure Assessment/Care

A. Monopolar Electrosurgery/Argon Plasma Coagulation
1. Patients with an implanted cardioverter-defibrillator (ICD) should have the device deactivated by a trained practitioner (RN), anesthesiologist or a cardiologist prior to the use of electrocautery devices. Deactivation may entail either temporary interruption via a "magnet" or actual shut off of device. With actual deactivation, the specialized personnel must remain present for transcutaneous control, monitoring, reactivation and assessment for normal device functioning throughout the entire procedural process.
2. Pre-procedural planning/assessement for patients with Pacemakers and/or ICDs includes knowledge of cardiac device make, model, type; indications for device, degree of pacemaker dependence and patient's underlying heart rhythm; in addition, for ICD patients, a history of device use is helpful.
3. For patients with non-cardiac implanted devices such as neurostimulators or implanted infusion pumps, seek proper guidance from physician specialist managing the device, as well as the manufacturer.

B. Bipolar Coagulation
Same as Flexible Bronchoscopy.

Patient Teaching

A. Monopolar Electrosurgery/Argon Plasma Coagulation
1. Explain the presence of the patient return electrode.
2. Avoid patient contact with metal side rails or other metal objects during use.
3. Explain to patient why removal of any jewelry is necessary, particularly safety aspects: inadvertent injury to patient by transfer of electrical current, or during emergent intubation.

B. Bipolar Coagulation
1. Same as Flexible Bronchoscopy.

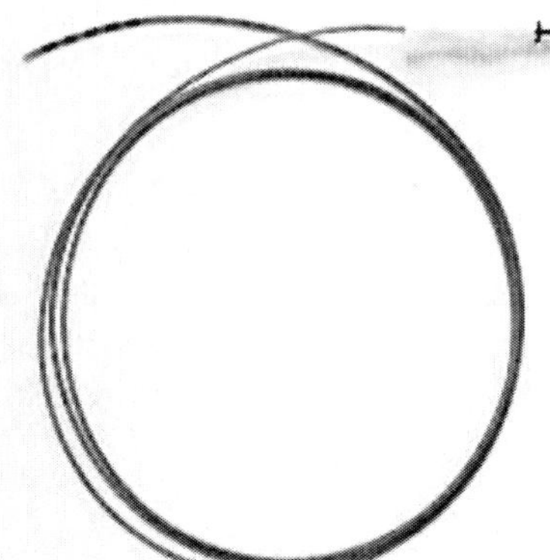

Figure 8: Argon plasma coagulator probe [Illustration courtesy of ERBE USA, Inc.]

Equipment

NOTE: Therapeutic bronchoscope is required to accommodate the accessories to be used (minimum of 2.6 mm channel).

A. Monopolar Electrosurgery
   1. Electrosurgical generator, monopolar output
   2. Patient return electrode (grounding pad)
   3. Active cord
   4. Snare, hot biopsy forceps or other electrosurgical accessories
   5. Disposable razor

B. Bipolar Coagulation
   1. Bipolar Unit
   2. Probe
   3. Sterile water and bottle for each particular unit
   4. To test probe – glass slide and normal saline for bipolar probe
   5. Gauze pads or alcohol to cleanse tip of probe

C. Argon Plasma Coagulation (APC)
   1. An argon capable electrosurgical generator with cables and foot pedal
   2. APC unit
   3. Argon gas source
   4. Endoscopic APC probe of appropriate size
   5. Cables
   6. Patient return electrodes (split pads recommended; do not use single pads because the built-in safety system of the APC unit cannot fully protect the patient)
   7. Gas filter; newest probes have the filter built into the probe;

Responsibilities During Procedure

A. Monopolar Electrosurgery/Argon Plasma Coagulation

NOTE: When argon is being used, it is essential that the nurse or associate visually and verbally verify that supplemental oxygen is turned off prior to and during each firing of the APC probe. (Per documented experience of physicians, supplemental O_2 concentration should be maintained at a minimum safe level; i.e., 40% or less for mechanically ventilated patients. Nasal cannula delivery is 3 liters/minute or less; Mask delivery of O_2 is to be avoided. Additionally, individual hospital policy and procedure should be followed regarding use of APC, as well as manufacturer's evidenced based recommendations.)

1. Apply the patient return electrode (grounding pad) according to the manufacturer's specifications observing the following guidelines:
   - Place the patient return electrode on a well-vascularized area of the body (such as the lower back or thigh) as close as possible to the operating field with the long edge of the rectangular plates facing the operating site.

   Especially for Children:

   Use pediatric grounding pad as needed. The child's upper thigh may not provide enough skin surface for proper application of a grounding plate. In these cases, the low back area may be used safely and effectively when electrocautery is anticipated.

   - The following placement sites should be avoided:
     - bony or uneven surfaces
     - hairy surfaces (may require shaving site for good contact of skin with entire electrode surface)
     - areas of high resistance such as areas with thick layers of fat (buttocks or stomach) or scar tissue

- **Position the patient return electrode so that that the flow of current is directed away from the pacemaker and does not pass through the area near the pacemaker.**
  NOTE: Patients with cardiac pacemakers have an increased risk of pacemaker malfunction or damage when electrosurgical units are used. Ask for advice from qualified cardiology staff or the manufacturer if in doubt of appropriate precautions to be taken.

2. Do not turn the power on until the physician is ready to use the electrosurgical unit, or use the "hold" or "standby" modes if available.
3. Follow the manufacturer's guidelines for equipment set-up.
4. Place foot pedal in the appropriate position for the physician.
5. Verify with the physician the mode desired (coagulation, cut or blend) and repeat settings.
6. Verbally confirm each setting change.
7. Document power settings per institution policy.
8. If electrical current is not conducted, check unit and all connections for secure fitting. Patient return electrode may need to be replaced for better contact.
9. Reassure and encourage the patient, keeping him as still as possible. Currently, many patients being treated with electrocautery/APC during bronchoscopy are intubated.
10. If electrical interference is noted with video endoscopy equipment, use appropriate grounding procedures recommended by manufacturer.

B. Bipolar Coagulation
1. Remind the physician to advance the probe with slow strokes to prevent possible kinking, which may break internal conduction wires.
2. Maintain the water level in the water bottle by adding sterile water.
3. Set the energy levels and water pressure as designated by the physician.
4. Wipe the probe with gauze as it is withdrawn from the scope to remove secretions.
5. Clean the probe tip as needed during the procedure.

Potential Complications

Same as Flexible Bronchoscopy

A. Monopolar Electrosurgery/Argon Plasma Coagulation
1. Endobronchial fire
2. Thermal injury to the patient
3. Malfunction of pacemaker or automatic implantable defibrillator
4. Hemorrhage
5. Perforation
6. Transmural burns
7. Explosion
8. Suffocation of patient and/or staff due to excessive argon inhalation
9. Gas embolism

B. Bipolar Cautery
1. Perforation
2. Delayed hemorrhage

Post-Procedure Assessment/Care

A. Monopolar Electrosurgery/Argon Plasma Coagulation
1. Same as Flexible Bronchoscopy or Rigid Bronchoscopy.
2. Check for skin damage or burns near and under the grounding pad.

B. Bipolar Coagulation
1. Same as Flexible Bronchoscopy, or Rigid Bronchoscopy, depending on procedure type.

References

American Society for Gastrointestinal Endoscopy. (2007). Endoscopy in patients with implanted electronic devices. *Gastrointestinal Endoscopy,* 65(4), 561-568.

Coulter, T. D., & Menta, A. C. (2000). The heat is on: Impact of endobronchial electrosurgery on the need for Nd-YAG laser photoresection. *Chest,* 118, 516-521.

ERBE. (2005). Using Argon Plasma Coagulation in Flexible Endoscopy: nurse self-study activity. (computer software). Denver: Healthstream.

Mourice, R. (2005). APC – Clinical Experiences in Interventional Bronchoscopy. (computer software) Denver. Retrieved from ERBE 11/2/06.

Binmoeller, K. (2005). APC – Clinical Applications. (computer software). Denver. Retrieved from ERBE 11/2/06.

Schonfeld, N., Temme, T., Serke, M., & Loddenkemper, R. (1999). High frequency diathermy--a new method in the treatment of malignant and benign stenosis of the airways. *Pneumologie,* 53, 477-9.

Sheski, F. D., & Mathur, P. N. (2000). Endoscopic treatment of early-stage lung cancer. *Cancer Control, 7* (1).

Ton, J. M., Westerga, J., Venmans, B. J. W., Postmus, P. E., & Sutedja, T. C. (2000). Tissue effects of bronchoscopic electrocautery. Bronchoscopic appearance and histologic changes of bronchial wall after electrocautery. *Chest,* 117, 887-891.

Foreign Body Removal

[Use in conjunction with Flexible Bronchoscopy, page 1, or Rigid Bronchoscopy, page 11]

Description

Foreign bodies may be removed from the respiratory tract using either the flexible bronchoscope or the rigid bronchoscope. The rigid bronchoscope is the instrument of choice in children. The flexible bronchoscope is the instrument of choice in adults, but either can be used in both populations, depending on the case. A variety of instruments may be used to retrieve foreign bodies dependent upon the type of matter involved.

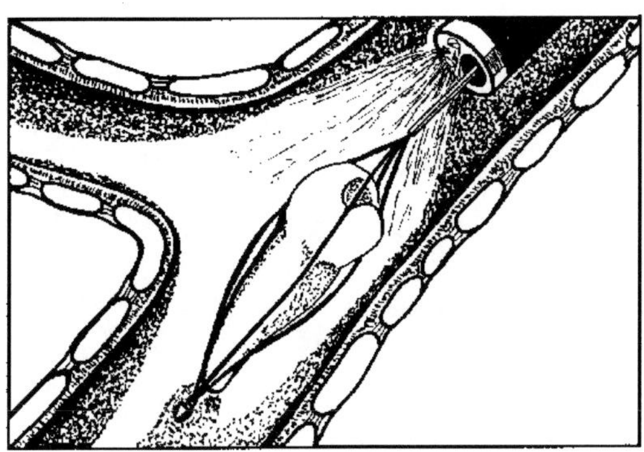

Figure 9: Foreign body in retrieval basket

Indications

1. Foreign body in airway

Contraindications

Contraindications describe circumstances in which a particular procedure is not usually performed. In some circumstances, however, the needs of the patient may require that a procedure proceed despite the presence of the condition. The physician makes these decisions.

1. Same as Flexible or Rigid Bronchoscopy
2. In rigid bronchoscopy, disease or trauma involving skull, jaw or cervical spine
3. Uncooperative patient

Especially for Children:

All procedures are contraindicated in the uncooperative or difficult to sedate patient. This becomes an important safety issue when upper endoscopy is applied for the purpose of foreign body removal, secondary to possible displacement of the foreign body into the airway. Very young or neurologically-handicapped children often do not have the ability to protect their airways in a normal fashion. Many institutions have adopted a policy to always use general anesthesia for foreign body removal in these children.

Pre-Procedure Assessment/Care

1. Same as Flexible or Rigid Bronchoscopy.
2. Obtain history and description of the foreign body, i.e., type of foreign body, location, length of time lodged, type and location of pain, previous X-rays, history of dysphagia, previous foreign body removal or other pertinent history or symptoms.

Patient Teaching

Same as Flexible or Rigid Bronchoscopy.

Equipment

1. If using flexible bronchoscope, refer to Flexible Bronchoscopy, page 1.
2. If using rigid bronchoscope, refer to Rigid Bronchoscopy, page 11.
3. Foreign bodies are removed with devices appropriate to the size, shape and consistency of the material. The following should be available for use:
    a. grasping forceps – alligator forceps, pronged grasping hooks
    b. baskets
    c. balloon catheters, such as a Fogarty catheter
    d. magnets
4. Magill forceps
5. If available, cryotherapy can be used.

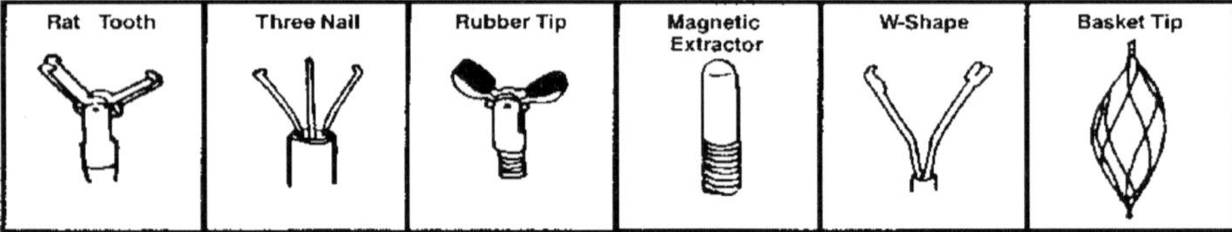

Figure 10: Retrieval instruments

Responsibilities During Procedure

1. Same as Flexible or Rigid Bronchoscopy.
2. Assist with elective intubation, if needed.
3. Assist physician during procedure passing instruments/accessories necessary for removal of the foreign body.
4. Properly handle, preserve, and label all specimens obtained. Removed foreign bodies may need to be identified by the laboratory per institutional policies.
5. Be aware that tracheostomy or further intervention may be necessary if airway becomes obstructed.
6. A combination of rigid and flexible bronchoscopes may be used to remove small, more distal fragments of a foreign body.

Potential Complications

1. Same as Flexible or Rigid Bronchoscopy
2. Displacement of foreign body to a more unfavorable or peripheral location
3. Fracture of an organic foreign body
4. Loss of a large foreign body in the subglottic area during withdrawal, resulting in airway obstruction

Post Procedure Assessment/Care

1. Same as Flexible or Rigid Bronchoscopy.
2. If patient has received general anesthesia, observe level of consciousness, character of respirations, movement of extremities, color and vital signs.

References

Boyd, M., Chatterjee, A., Chiles, C., Chin, R. (2009).Tracheobronchial Foreign Body Aspiration in Adults. *Southern Medical Journal*, 102, (2), 171-174.

Fairchild, S. (1996). *Perioperative nursing, principles and practice* (2nd ed.). Boston: Little, Brown.

Fishman, A., Elias, J., Fishman, J., & Grippi, M. (2008). *Fishman's Pulmonary diseases and disorders* (4th ed.). New York: McGraw-Hill.

Kneedler, J. A., & Dodge, G. (1994). *Perioperative patient care, the nursing perspective.* Boston: Jones and Barlett.

Mason, R., Broaddus, V., Murray, J., & Nadel, J. (Eds). (2005). *Textbook of Respiratory Medicine* (4th ed.), (vol. 1). Philadelphia: W.B. Saunders.

Rothrock, J. C. (1996). *Perioperative nursing care planning.* St. Louis: Mosby.

Wang, K., & Mehta, A. C. (2012). *Flexible bronchoscopy* (3rd ed.). Cambridge, MA: Blackwell Science.

Laser (Photocoagulation/Vaporization) Therapy

[Use in conjunction with Flexible Bronchoscopy, page 1]

Description

Laser is an acronym for Light Amplification by Stimulated Emission of Radiation. Currently, Argon and Nd:YAG (Neodymium-Yttrium-Aluminum-Garnet) lasers are used in endoscopy. The light energy is transmitted through a quartz fiber catheter (fiber), which can be passed through a flexible endoscope. The laser fiber is designed with an external catheter to provide air/gas flow; carbon dioxide may be used. The adjustable gas flow rate is designed to help clear the treatment area of blood and debris as well as help protect the laser fiber from overheating. The gas can be retrieved by suctioning through the scope or by a gas retrieval system built into the laser. Repeated laser treatments are frequently necessary.

Indications

1. Benign or malignant tumors of the bronchial tree unresponsive to conventional therapies
2. Hemorrhagic conditions of the respiratory tract requiring hemostasis

Contraindications

Contraindications describe circumstances in which a particular procedure is not usually performed. In some circumstances, however, the needs of the patient may require that a procedure proceed despite the presence of the condition. The physician makes these decisions.

1. Same as Flexible Bronchoscopy
2. Extremely large vessel in the field
3. Inaccessible lesion

Pre-Procedure Assessment/Care

Same as Flexible Bronchoscopy

Patient Teaching

1. Same as Flexible Bronchoscopy
2. Explain to the outpatient the possibility of admission to the hospital after the procedure

Equipment

1. Refer to manufacturer's guidelines
2. Biopsy forceps
3. Hydrogen peroxide
4. Laser with ancillary equipment
5. Laser fiber with back-up fiber
6. CO_2 tank
7. Safety glasses or goggles for every person in the room, including the patient
8. Filtering lens for bronchoscope if necessary
9. "Laser in Use" signs for all entrances to the laser room
10. High filtration mask
11. Smoke evacuator

    NOTE: Smoke emitted from tumor vaporization may contain carcinogens. All personnel should wear masks to prevent inhalation of smoke.
12. Fire extinguisher / basin of saline or water
13. Documentation tools: laser pre- and post-procedure safety check lists and log sheet with patient data for future procedure reference

Responsibilities During Procedure

1. Same as Flexible Bronchoscopy.
2. Display warning signs, close doors, cover windows and give protective glasses or goggles and masks to everyone in the room.
3. Maintain laser in standby mode when laser not in firing position.
4. Calibrate fiber and set power and duration desired by physician.
5. Clean fiber tip with hydrogen peroxide as needed.
6. Assist physician with biopsy forceps for possible debridement of treatment site.

Potential Complications

1. Same as Flexible Bronchoscopy
2. Tissue sloughing
3. Perforation
4. Ulceration
5. Delayed healing
6. Fistula formation

Post-Procedure Assessment/Care

1. Same as Flexible Bronchoscopy.
2. Reassure the patient that it is normal to have discomfort at the treatment site; patient may need medication.
3. Admit the patient to the hospital if ordered by physician. Because of the laser's thermal effect, tissue and airway edema may be present.

Special Considerations

1. Refer to *Safety* (see page 87) and *Standard Equipment* (see pages 95).
2. If laser treatment is done through a rigid bronchoscope, the patient should receive general anesthesia. The OR and institutional laser safety policies should be followed.
3. It is very important to have an institutional policy for laser procedure. Clearly detailed procedures and policies should include safety, equipment operation and maintenance, personnel training and scheduling.

References

Allard, D. (1993). Defining performance expectations for laser nurses and technicians. *Clinical Laser Monthly*, 11(2), 12-15.

Buszta, C., & Sovero, B. S. (1994). Developing laser competencies: A process to ensure safe practice. *AORN Journal*, 59, 467-471.

Sheski, F. D., & Mathur, P. N. (2001). Endoscopic options in the management of airway obstruction. In R. B. George & G. B. Epler (Eds.). *Pulmonary and critical care update on-line, 14* (lesson 21) [On-line]. Available: http://www.chestnet.org/education/pccu/vol14/lesson21-22.index.html.

Thomas, S. and Mathew, A. (2002). Therapeutic Bronchial Laser Resection and Airway Stenting. *Gastroenterology Nursing*, 25(2), 60-65.

Photodynamic Therapy (PDT)

[Use in conjunction with Flexible Bronchoscopy, page 1]

Description

Photodynamic therapy (PDT) is one specific method in which laser is used to kill cancer cells. A photosensitizing agent that concentrates especially within malignant tissue is injected 2 to 3 days prior to the procedure. The malignant area is then exposed to laser light energy and the sensitizing agent causes the production of singlet oxygen, which damages the cancer cells. PDT can be used for early-staged lung cancer, and if used for carcinoma in situ, remission rate is high. Photodynamic Therapy is a two-step process which uses a combination of a photoactive drug (a drug that is activated by light), and a specific frequency of light from a laser. Both work together to allow the physician to specifically target and destroy cancer cells while limiting damage to surrounding healthy tissue.

Indications

1. Laryngeal cancer
2. Lung cancer
3. Tracheal cancer

Contraindications

Contraindications describe circumstances in which a particular procedure is not usually performed. In some circumstances, however, the needs of the patient may require that a procedure proceed despite the presence of the condition. The physician makes these decisions.

1. Patients with porphyria or with known allergies to porphyrins
2. Patients with an existing tracheoesophageal or bronchoesophageal fistula
3. Patients with tumors eroding into major blood vessels
4. Caution must be given to patients receiving other photosensitizing agents

Pre-procedure Assessment/Care

1. Same as Flexible Bronchoscopy.
2. Verify informed consent specific to PDT.
3. Screen patients for porphyria or allergies to porphyrins.
4. Confirm the patient has not received radiotherapy for four weeks prior to PDT treatment and that radiotherapy will not commence for two to four weeks post-PDT therapy.
5. Keep the patient covered to prevent inadvertent sensitization from the therapeutic light.
6. Avoid exposure to bright light.
   NOTE: Photofrin is administered intravenously 40 to 50 hours prior to laser light treatment. Patient/caregiver education covering photosensitivity precautions must be completed before drug administration. Patients remain photosensitive for 30 days.

Patient Teaching

1. Same as Flexible Bronchoscopy.
2. Explain to the patient/family members that the procedure may take several hours.
3. If the patient will be an inpatient post-procedure, review the special considerations in caring for photosensitive patients with the inpatient nurse.
4. Review with patient/caregiver the photosensitivity precautions for outdoors.
   a. sunscreens offer no protection
   b. long-sleeved shirt, jacket dark in color, long pants
   c. gloves and a hat with a brim to cover ears and forehead
   d. sunglasses with maximum UV protection

   e. when riding in an automobile during daylight hours, wear protective clothing
5. Review with patient/caregiver the photosensitivity precautions for indoors.
   a. avoid sitting near bright unshaded windows during daylight hours
   b. avoid sitting close to unshaded light bulbs (e.g., directly under a reading lamp)
   c. avoid bright exam lights (similar to dental or eye exam lights)
   d. it is not necessary to keep the house dark; ambient light indoors is helpful in ridding the body of the drug
6. Patients will remain photosensitive for 30 days. Afterwards, gradually expose skin to daylight (in 10-minute increments). If photosensitivity reactions occur (such as edema and blistering), continue photosensitivity precautions for an additional 2 weeks.

Equipment

1. Same as Flexible Bronchoscopy
2. Proper laser signs (to be put on door)
3. Appropriate eyewear
4. Fire extinguisher
5. Basin of saline or water
6. PDT dye module with KTP pump laser
7. PDT fiber

Responsibilities During Procedure

1. Same as Flexible Bronchoscopy.
2. Know institution's policy and procedure on laser use.
3. Insure that patient and all staff are wearing laser safety glasses prior to laser activation.

Potential Complications

1. Tumor hemorrhage
2. Substernal chest pain
3. Photosensitivity reactions

Post Procedure Assessment/Care

1. Same as Flexible Endoscopy
2. Follow photosensitivity precautions including posting a sign above patient's bed.
3. Notify patient of potential for substernal chest pain due to inflammatory process, which may require short-term opiates.
4. Provide written soft diet instructions.
5. Schedule follow-up endoscopy procedure in two days for potential tumor debridement.
6. Review photosensitivity instructions.

NOTE: Repeat courses of Photofrin may be administered at 30-day intervals with a maximum total of three courses.

References

Axcan Pharma, Inc. *Photofrin® Frequently Asked Questions*. (2008). Axcan Pharma, Inc. Retrieved on Feb. 3, 2012 from http://photofrin.com/faqs.

Diaz-Jimenez, J., Martinex-Ballarin, J., Llunell, A., Farrero, E., Rodriguez, A., & Castro, M. (1999). Efficacy and safety of photodynamic therapy versus Nd-YAG laser resection in NSCLC with airway obstruction. *European Respiratory Journal,* 14, 800-805.

Dougherty, T., Gomer, C., Henderson, B., Jori, G., Kessel, D., Korbelik, M., Moan, J., & Peng, Q. (1998). Photodynamic therapy review. *Journal of the National Cancer Institute,* 90, 889-905.

Kato, H. (1998). Photodynamic therapy for lung cancer – A review of 19 years' experience. *Journal of Photochemistry and Photobiology B,* 42, 96-99.

Maziak DE, Markman RB, MacKay JA et al. (2004). Photodynamic Therapy in nonsmall cell lung cancer : a systemic review. *Ann Thoracic Surgery*, 77, 1484.

Speer, C. (2006). A Photodynamic Therapy for Ampullary Cancer. *Gastroenterology Nursing*, 29, 398-400.

Tracheobronchial Stents

[Use in conjunction with Flexible Bronchoscopy, page 1 or Rigid Bronchoscopy, page 11]

Description

Tracheobronchial stents are placed into the airway to maintain patency of the respiratory tract. Stents are made from several different materials and are available in a vast variety of sizes and shapes. The main classes of stents available are silicone, metal and hybrid stents.

Indications

1. Occlusion of airway secondary to malignant neoplasm
   a. primary or metastatic lung cancer with extrinsic compression
   b. following debulking of bronchogenic lesions
2. Occlusion of airway secondary to benign conditions
   a. traumatic injury - post intubation
   b. post-transplant stricture
   c. post infectious scarring or stricture
   d. in conjunction with esophageal stent for tracheoesophageal fistula
   e. benign tumors

Contraindications

Contraindications describe circumstances in which a particular procedure is not usually performed. In some circumstances, however, the needs of the patient may require that a procedure proceed despite the presence of the condition. The physician makes these decisions.

1. Same as Flexible or Rigid Bronchoscopy
2. Obstructions that cannot be opened and maintained to 4mm - sufficient size to pass and allow expansion of stent
3. Conditions where less aggressive therapy is still available
4. Prior to laser therapy, endobronchial electrocautery or argon plasma coagulation

Pre-Procedure Assessment/Care

Same as Flexible or Rigid Bronchoscopy

Patient Teaching

Same as Flexible or Rigid Bronchoscopy

Equipment

1. Same as Flexible or Rigid Bronchoscopy
2. Stent (selection generally determined during previous bronchoscopy)
   a. types: solid or mesh
   b. material: metal or plastic
3. Guidewire
4. Dilation equipment (optional)
5. Fluoroscopy and radiation protection for staff and patient

NOTE: If using laser or other debulking modalities, refer to appropriate procedures and institutional policies.

Responsibilities During Procedure

1. Same as Flexible or Rigid Bronchoscopy.

Therapeutic Pulmonary Procedures

2. Assist physician during procedure passing instruments/accessories necessary to debulk tumor.
3. Assist in measuring the distance from the vocal cord to the lesion, the length of the lesion and the diameter of the lesion to aide in the selection of the stent.
4. Assist with deployment of the stent; have grasping devices available for manipulation of the stent for optimal placement.

Potential Complications

1. Same as Flexible or Rigid Bronchoscopy.
2. Most airway stents are well tolerated. Complications can occur, but serious life threatening complications are rare.
3. Stent migration.
4. Occlusion of airway from granuloma, tumor regrowth or impaction/accumulated respiratory secretions.
5. Airway wall perforation.
6. Stent wire failure.

Post-Procedure Assessment/Care

Same as Flexible or Rigid Bronchoscopy

References

Dumon, J-F., & Dumon, M. C. (2000). Dumon-Novatech Y-stents: A four-year experience with 50 tracheobronchial tumors involving the carina. *Journal of Bronchology, 7*, 26-32.

Mehta, A. C., & Dasgupta, A. (1999). Airway stents. *Clinics in Chest Medicine, 20*, 139-151.

Nesbitt, J. C., & Carrasco, H. (1996). Expandable stents. *Chest Surgery Clinics in North America, 6*, 305-328.

Sheski, F. D., & Mathur, P. N. (2001). Endoscopic options in the management of airway obstruction. In R. B. George & G. B. Epler (Eds.), *Pulmonary and critical care update on-line, 14* (lesson 21) [On-line]. Available: http://www.chestnet.org/education/pccu/vol14/lesson21-22.index.html.

Ranu, H & Madden, BP. (2009). Endobronchial Stenting in the management of the large airway Pathology. *PostGra Medical Journal*, 85, 682.

Bronchial Thermoplasty

[Use in conjunction with Flexible Bronchoscopy, page 1]

Description

Bronchial thermoplasty (BT) is an outpatient procedure designed to help control asthma by reducing the mass of airway smooth muscle (ASM). Thermal energy is delivered to the airway wall, heating the tissue in a controlled manner in order to reduce ASM mass. Reducing ASM is believed to decrease muscle-mediated bronchoconstriction, thereby reducing asthma symptoms and exacerbations. Bronchial thermoplasty is expected to compliment asthma maintenance medications as an add-on therapy that decreases morbidity associated with severe asthma. In fact, bronchial thermoplasty has been demonstrated to reduce the number and percent of subjects with severe exacerbations and emergency room visits for respiratory symptoms, as well as reduce time lost from work, school and other daily activities due to asthma symptoms.

Indications

1. Adult severe, persistent asthmatics (≥ 18 years old) with inadequate control despite combination of inhaled high dose corticosteroids (ICS) and a long-acting beta-agonists (LABA).
2. Patient must be able to safely undergo bronchoscopy per hospital guidelines.

Contraindications

Contraindications describe circumstances in which a particular procedure is not usually performed. In some circumstances, however, the needs of the patient may require that a procedure proceed despite the presence of the condition. The physician makes these decisions.

1. Patients with an active implantable electronic device.
2. Known sensitivity to medications used in bronchoscopy.
3. Previously treated airways of the lung should not be retreated with the Alair® Bronchial Thermoplasty System.
4. Patients who are not stable and suitable to undergo bronchoscopy.

Pre-Procedure Assessment/Care

1. Patient evaluated 1 week prior to procedure to verify ability to undergo bronchoscopy.
2. Prophylactic oral corticoidsteroids (OCS) initiated 3 days prior, day of and day after procedure.
3. Lung function evaluated morning of procedure to assess stability.

:

Patient Teaching

Same as Flexible Bronchoscopy.

Equipment

1. Same as Flexible Bronchoscopy.
2. Alair® Catheter - A single-use device designed to be delivered through the working channel of a standard bronchoscope.
3. Alair® Radiofrequency (RF) Controller - Designed with a proprietary set of control parameters and algorithms to deliver the correct intensity and duration of thermal energy sufficient to reduce the mass of ASM tissue, while limiting long-term impact to surrounding tissues.
4. A grounding pad.

Responsibilities During Procedure

1. Same as Flexible Bronchoscopy.
2. Albuterol and an antisialogogue agent administered 30 minutes before the start of the procedure.
3. BT catheter introduced through flexible bronchoscope and RF energy applied to airways (approx. 60 activations per procedure).
4. Each procedure completed within 40-60 minutes.

Potential Complications

1. Same as Flexible Bronchoscopy
2. Expected transient increase in the frequency and worsening of respiratory-related symptoms
3. Hemoptysis
4. Fever, cough
5. Sinusitis
6. Headache
7. Throat pain
8. Chest pain

Post-Procedure Assessment/Care

1. Patient monitored for 2-4 hours post-op
2. Patient discharged from hospital same day
3. Lung function stable within 80% of the pre-procedure post bronchodilator forced expiratory volume in 1 second (BD FEV1)
4. Patient stable, able to take liquids, feeling well, adequate mental status
5. Prophylactic OCS (oral corticosteroids) continued 1 day after procedure
6. Patient contacted via phone at 1, 2 and 7 days to assess post procedure status
7. Office visit at 2 to 3 weeks to assess clinical stability and schedule subsequent BT procedures as appropriate
8. Individual patient results are communicated to referring physician as appropriate
9. Patient returns to care of primary asthma physician for long term asthma management following BT

References

Castro M, et al. (2010). Effectiveness and Safety of Bronchial Thermoplasty in the Treatment of Severe Asthma: A Multicenter, Randomized, Double-Blind, Sham-Controlled Clinical Trial. *American Journal of Respiratory & Critical Care Medicine*, 181, 116-124. Retrieved on Jan. 21, 2012 from http://ajrccm.atsjournals.org/cgi/reprint/181/2/116.pdf

Castro M, et al. (2011). Persistence of Effectiveness of Bronchial Thermoplasty in Patients with Severe Asthma. *Annals of Asthma, Allergy and Immunology*, 107(1), 65-70. Retrieved on Jan. 21, 2012 from http://www.cenveomobile.com/issue/35148.

Cox G, et al. (2007). Asthma Control During the Year After Bronchial Thermoplasty. *New England Journal of Medicine*, 356, 1327-1337. Retrieved on Jan. 22, 2012 from www.nejm.org/doi/pdf/10.1056/NEJMoa064707.

Cox G, et al. (2006). Bronchial Thermoplasty for Asthma. *American Journal of Respiratory & Critical Care Medicine* , 173, 965-969. Retrieved on January 22, 2012 from http://ajrccm.atsjournals.org/cgi/reprint/173/9/965.pdf.

Danek, CJ, et al. (2004). Reduction in airway hyperresponsiveness to methacholine by the application of RF energy in dogs. *Journal of Applied Physiology*, 97, 1946-1953. Retrieved on Jan. 21, 2012 from http://jap.physiology.org/content/97/5/1946.full.pdf+html.

Duhamel DR, Hales JB. (2010). Bronchial Thermoplasty: A Novel Therapeutic Approach to Severe Asthma. *JoVE*, 45. Retrieved on Jan. 21, 2012 from www.jove.com/details.php?id=2428.

Mayse M, et al. (2007). Clinical Pearls for Bronchial Thermoplasty. *Journal of Bronchology*, 14, 115-123. Retrieved on January 18, 2012 from http://delivery.sheridan.com/downloads/mobile/SAGE_168664_CP.exe.

Pavord I, et al. (2007). Safety and Efficacy of Bronchial Thermoplasty in Symptomatic Severe Asthma. American Journal of Respiratory & Critical Care Medicine 2007; 176: 1185-1191. Retrieved on January 18, 2012 from http://ajrccm.atsjournals.org/cgi/reprint/176/12/1185.pdf.

Thomson N, et al. (2011). Long-term (5 year) Safety of Bronchial Thermoplasty: Asthma Intervention Research (AIR) Trial, BMC Medicine. Retrieved on January 21, 2012 from www.biomedcentral.com/content/pdf/1471-2466-11-8.pdf.

Wilson S, et al. (2006). Global assessment after bronchial thermoplasty: the patient's perspective. *Journal of Outcomes Research*, 10, 37-46.

Video Intubation Scopes

[Use in conjunction with Flexible Bronchoscopy, page 1]

Description

Video intubation scopes provide verifiable glottic exposure and decrease risks of difficult intubation.

Flexible tracheal intubation fiberscopes can be used with Xenon lightsource, Halogen lightsource or a miniature battery powered lightsource. These have a range of diameters enabling insertion through an endotracheal tube and have a suction channel to allow suctioning during intubation.

Videolaryngoscopes are used similar in technique to direct laryngoscopy. The videolaryngoscope has a blade and handle like a normal laryngoscope. The image is captured by a miniature camera embedded in the blade and visualized on the monitor attached to a video cable from the handle.

Indications

1. Anticipated difficult intubations by history or physical exam

Pre-Procedure Assessment and Care

1. Same as Flexible Bronchoscopy

Patient Teaching

1. Determine the patient's readiness to learn and level of knowledge.
2. Explain the purpose of the procedure, the positioning and techniques to be used.
3. Explain the purpose of all the equipment that is used.
4. Explain the need and rationale for the supplemental administration of oxygen during the exam.
5. Explain the effects of and rationale for the medications used and their methods of administration.

Equipment/Supplies

1. Appropriately sized intubation tube
2. Light source, video imaging system
3. Two suction sources
4. Monitoring system which includes blood pressure, oxygen levels, capnography (facility specfic) and cardiac rhythms
5. Oxygen and delivery device (e.g., cannula, catheter, face mask)
6. Medications to administer per physician discretion
7. Intravenous supplies
8. Emergency airway equipment
9. Emergency medication box

Responsibilities During Procedure

1. Assist physician as needed.

Potential Complications

1. Hypoxemia
2. Bronchospasm
3. Cardiac dysrhythmias

4. Respiratory and/or cardiac arrest
5. Laryngospasm
6. Hypoventilation
7. Laryngeal edema and/or injury

Post-Procedure Assessment/Care

Same as for extubated patient

References

Aziz, M. F., Dillman, D., Fu, R. and Brambrink, A. (2012). Comparative effectiveness of the C-MAC video laryngoscope versus direct laryngoscopy in the setting of the predicted difficult airway. *Anesthesiology*, 116(3), 629-636.

Cooper, R. M. (2003). Use of a new videolaryngoscope (GlideScope) in the management of a difficult airway. *Canadian Journal of Anesthesia*. 50(6), 611-613.

PortaView-LF Tracheal Intubation Fiberscope Olympus LF-GP/TP/DP Olympus America. Retrieved on March 17, 2012 from http://www.olympusamerica.com/msg_section/download_brochures/DPTPGP_SalesLiterature.pdf.

Part 3

SPECIMEN COLLECTION

Arterial Blood Gases Sampling

Description

Arterial blood gas (ABG) analysis is one way of monitoring lung function and the primary means of assessing acid/base balance. It can help differentiate between respiratory acid/base disorders vs. metabolic acid/base disorders and guide treatment.

Glossary

1. Bicarbonate – a chemical buffer that helps keep the pH of the blood within normal limits.
2. Oxygen saturation – measurement of the amount of oxygen found in the blood. Low O_2 saturations may indicate decreased levels of oxygen in the air, COPD, pneumonia, heart failure, pulmonary edema, pulmonary emboli or hypoventilation.

Indications

1. Evaluate respiratory status
2. Evaluate response to therapy
3. Monitor progression of respiratory disorders
4. Evaluate for presence and type of acid-base disorders

Contraindications

Contraindications describe circumstances in which a particular procedure is not usually performed. In some circumstances, however, the needs of the patient may require that a procedure proceed despite the presence of the condition. The physician makes these decisions.

1. Failure to show good collateral circulation to hand (absolute)
2. Absence of palpable radial pulse
3. Sign of infection, cellulitis or open wounds, or fractures near chosen site
4. On anticoagulation therapy such as heparin or warfarin (Coumadin™) (relative)
5. Inability to transport ABG specimen to lab in timely and appropriate manner (this may be of important consideration in an off-site clinic or lab) (relative)

When not to get blood gases

1. When the results will not change therapy
2. Do not do if there is something less painful or less expensive that would give same information (pulse oximeter to evaluate for adequate oxygenation)

Sites of Sampling

1. Radial artery – most common puncture site
2. Dorsalis pedis artery
3. Brachial and femoral arteries – high risk of neurovascular injury, principal source of blood supply to extremity
4. Indwelling arterial cannula

Pre-Procedure Assessment

1. Radial site - Check for collateral circulation by having patient clench fist (Allen's Test). Compress radial and ulnar arteries. When patient opens hand the palm should be pale in color. When pressure over ulnar artery is released, normal color should return to palm within 1 to 2 seconds. If not, choose the other wrist or try brachial artery.
2. Obtain current temperature, hemoglobin and flow rate of supplemental oxygen.
3. These factors may interfere with the test and accuracy of the results:

A. a fever may raise the oxygen and carbon dioxide values; an abnormally low temperature may lower the values
B. severe anemia or polycythemia
C. smoking or being exposed to second hand smoke, or carbon monoxide may lower O_2 saturations without affecting partial pressure of O_2 ($PaCO_2$)
D. Air bubbles in the syringe
E. More than an hour since blood collected before test is run

Patient Teaching

1. Determine the patient's readiness to learn and level of knowledge.
2. Explain the purpose of the procedure, positioning, techniques to be used, and sensations a patient may experience during and after the procedure.
3. Explain that there may be some discomfort during insertionof the needle.
4. Call physician if signs of infection, numbness, tingling, excessive bleeding and/or weakness of extremity.
5. Leave dressing on for about 30 to 60 minutes.
6. Keep puncture site clean and protected until healed.
7. Document teaching and patient response.

Equipment

1. Arterial blood gas supplies (heparinized syringe, sterile needles, gauze, skin antiseptic swabs, rubber stopper or needle cap, adhesive bandage/tape)
2. Appropriate laboratory slip
3. Gloves
4. Container with ice if unable to get to lab within minutes
5. Optional: 1% lidocaine solution

Procedure

1. Check identity band, verify name and date of birth with patient.
2. Do teaching and answer questions.
3. Wash hands and put on gloves.
4. Choose appropriate arterial puncture site; radial is usually considered safer than brachial and has smaller risk of nerve injury. Perform Allen's test to check circulation.
5. Clean the insertion site with an antimicrobial swab using a circular motion per facilities policy. Allow to dry.
6. Consider local anesthetic at entry site.
7. Locate appropriate artery by palpating site with two fingers slightly apart.
8. Dorsiflex wrist to stabilize radial artery.
9. Insert needle at 45-degree angle. Gently advance until blood appears in the needle hub. Allow syringe to fill to appropriate level before withdrawing.
10. If flow ceases, slowly withdraw needle 1-2 mm to reposition needle back inside artery.
11. Apply direct pressure to insertion site for a full 5 minutes (longer if patient is on anticoagulation therapy). Apply dressing.
12. Expel all air from syringe, insert needle into cork (or other appropriate device), rotate specimen to mix blood with heparin.
13. Label specimen, and fill out lab form completely (per institution policy/procedure), place on ice and send to lab.
14. Check site for adequate perfusion and hematoma.
15. Record results of Allen's test, time drawn, patient's temperature, site of puncture, amount of time pressure applied and oxygen therapy.

Potential Complications

1. Arterial spasm may affect circulation to extremity
2. Hematoma
3. Site infection
4. Pain
5. Arterial occlusion or trauma
6. Nerve damage
7. Vasovagal response

Post-Procedure Assessment/Care

1. Evaluate puncture site for bleeding; maintain pressure on site until bleeding stops.
2. Assess peripheral pulses distal to the puncture site and document.
3. Keep the puncture site clean and protected until healed.

ABG Analysis

1. Decide if pH is normal or acidic/alkalotic.

pH		
< 7.35	7.35-7.45	> 7.45
Acidosis	Normal or Compensated	Alkalosis

2. Determine the respiratory effect.

$PaCO_2$ – The Respiratory Effect		
<35	35-45	>45
Tends toward alkalosis Causes high pH Neutralizes low pH	Normal or Compensated	Tends toward acidosis Causes low pH Neutralizes high pH

3. Evaluate the metabolic component.

HCO_3 – The Metabolic Component		
<22	22-26	>26
Acidosis	Normal or compensated	Alkalosis

Low pH		High pH	
Acidosis		Alkalosis	
High $PaCO_2$	Low $PaCO_2$	High $PaCO_2$	Low $PaCO_2$
Respiratory	Metabolic	Metabolic	Respiratory

References

Argyle, B. (1996). Blood Gases Computer Program Manual. (Mad Scientist Software) Alpine UT. Retrieved on Nov. 2, 2006 from http://www.madsci.com/manu/gas_gen.htm.

Emergency Nurses Association. (2007). *Trauma Nursing Core Course Provider Manual* (6th ed.). Des Plaines: Author.

Rn.com. (2011). Interpreting ABGs: The Basics. Retrieved on Jan. 15, 2012 from www.rn.com/getpdf.php/1670.pdf?Main_Session.

Smith, S.P., Duell, D.J., & Martin, B.C. (2004). *Clinical nursing skills: basic to advanced skills* (6th ed.). Upper Saddle River, NJ: Pearson Education Inc.

Springhouse. (2003). *Nursing Procedures & Protocols.* Philadelphia: Lippincott, Williams & Wilkins.

Ureden, L. D., Stacy, K. M., Lough, M. E. (2010). *Critical Care Nursing: Diagnosis and Management* (6th ed.). St. Louis: Mosby.

Woodruff, D. W. (2009). 6 Easy Steps to ABG Analysis. Retrieved on Jan, 15, 2012 from www.ed4nurses.com/resources/1/pdf/ABGebook.pdf.

Endobronchial and Transbronchial Biopsy

(Use in conjunction with Flexible Bronchoscopy, page 1)

Description

Using biopsy forceps during bronchoscopy, small tissue samples from the airway (endobronchial biopsy) or from the lung parenchyma (transbronchial biopsy) are obtained for microscopic examination. Tissue samples may be visual lesions or lesions that can only be seen by fluoroscope.

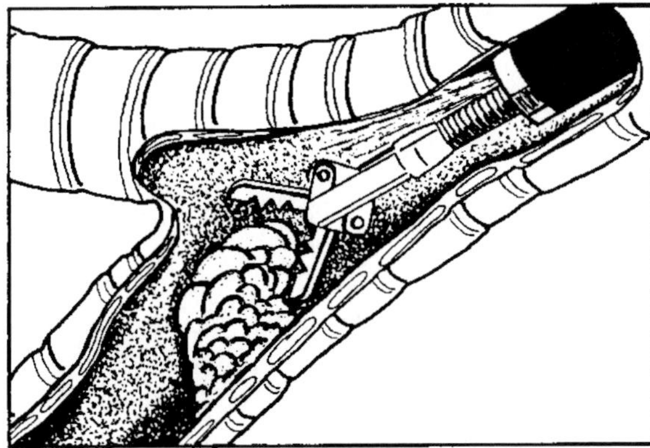

Figure 11: Endobronchial biopsy

Indications

1. Suspicion of abnormal tissue
2. Confirmation of normal tissue
3. Diagnosis of pulmonary infections

Contraindications

Contraindications describe circumstances in which a particular procedure is not usually performed. In some circumstances, however, the needs of the patient may require that a procedure proceed despite the presence of the condition. The physician makes these decisions.

1. Same as Flexible Bronchoscopy
2. Bleeding disorder
   a. coagulopathy (relative)
   b. active bleeding (relative)
   c. thrombocytopenia (absolute)
   d. current use of anticoagulants (relative)
3. Severe pulmonary hypertension (relative)
4. Recent ingestion of non-steroidal anti-inflammatory or aspirin – containing drugs (relative)
5. Suspected arteriovenous malformation (relative)
6. Patient's inability to control cough during procedure (relative)
7. Uncooperative patient (absolute)

Pre-Procedure Assessment and Care

1. Same as Flexible Bronchoscopy.
2. If procedure is to be done under fluoroscopy, ensure patient is secure with straps as needed and protected for fluoroscopy exposure. Metallic pads and wires should be arranged so they do not interfere with image to be biopsied.

Patient Teaching

1. Same as Flexible Bronchoscopy
2. Inform the patient that blood may be expected post biopsy
3. Pre-arrange communication sign for pain (hand gesture)
4. Signs of lung collapse

Equipment and Accessory Supplies

1. Same as Flexible Bronchoscopy
2. Chest tube set-up
3. Gauze sponges
4. Epinephrine

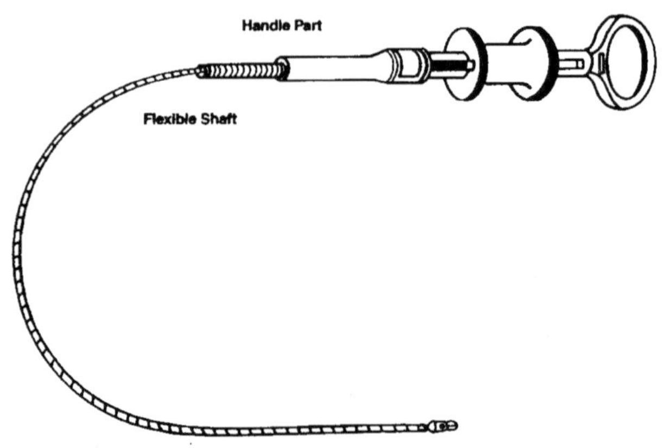

Figure 12: Biopsy forceps

Various Biopsy Forcep Tips

Standard Fenestrated — A
Ellipsoid Fenestrated — B
Fenestrated Ellipsoid w/Needle — C

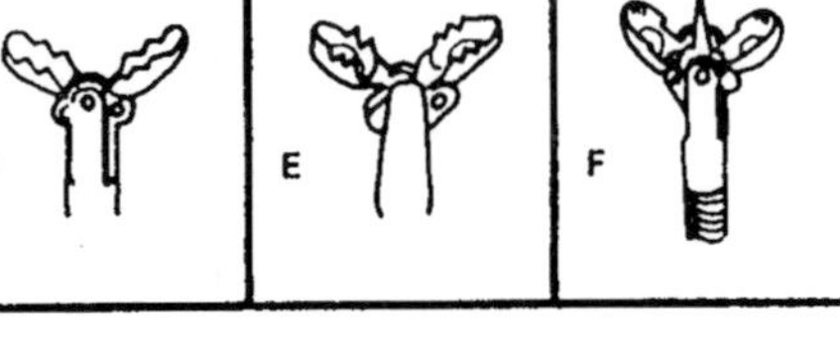

A. Round cups with side holes allow for clean biopsy with minimal tissue damage.
B. Oval cups for deeper biopsy.
C. Oval cups for deeper biopsy. Needle in center anchors forceps for more accurate biopsy of slippery tissue.
D. Serrated oval jaws for biopsy of tough tissue.
E. Serrated side for biopsy following laser procedure.
F. Needle in round cups with side holes allows for clean, accurate biopsy when targeting position is less than ideal.

Figure 13: Various biopsy forceps tips

Responsibilities During Procedure

Same as Flexible Bronchoscopy

Obtaining Endobronchial Biopsy

1. Cytology samples, brushings and washings should be obtained before biopsy of tissue.
2. Check forceps by opening and closing several times before insertion into the scope to verify proper operation.
3. Assist the physician in passing biopsy forceps, in closed position, through biopsy valve and down the endoscope channel.
4. Open and close forceps, at physician's request.
5. Withdraw forceps from the channel in the closed position, taking care not to dislodge the specimen.
6. When withdrawing the forceps, wipe shaft with a gauze sponge to remove secretions.
7. Prepare specimens as per institution policy.
8. Rinse the tip of the forceps with sterile saline after each use.
9. Inform the physician about the number and adequacy of the specimen obtained.

10. Alert the bronchoscopist to any grimacing or other indications of patient experiencing pain when the forceps are closed.
11. Place specimen in container with appropriate solution. NOTE: Place any specimens for culture in non-bacteriostatic saline.
12. Label the container with pertinent patient information, timing and site of the biopsy.
13. Confirm with the physician when a separate container should be used.
14. If bleeding occurs during biopsy, the physician determines assessment of the amount. Saline in 5-10cc increments may be instilled through the bronchoscope to assess the amount of bleeding. Epinephrine (1:1,000 diluted with normal saline to either 1:10,000 or 1:20,000) may be instilled onto the bleeding site to control bleeding. Subsequent saline wash may be instilled through the bronchoscope to re-assess the amount and/or control of bleeding.
15. If bleeding remains uncontrolled, prepare for emergency endotracheal intubation, use of tamponade balloon or IV administration of blood-clotting medications.
16. Position patient on side with unaffected lung up to prevent possible aspiration of blood into the unaffected lung.

Obtaining Transbronchial Biopsy (TRBB)

1. Follow the procedure as described above.
2. Fluoroscopy is frequently used when obtaining transbronchial tissue. The forceps are advanced through the bronchoscope beyond the tip into the peripheral area to be biopsied. After position is obtained under fluoroscopy, the forceps are withdrawn slightly, opened and then advanced until resistance is felt. If fluoroscopy was not used during TRBB, a chest x-ray should be obtained if shortness of breath, chest pain or coughing occurred during or after procedure.
3. The biopsy should be obtained during the exhalation phase to reduce the risk of pneumothorax.
4. Controversy exists regarding the number of biopsies to do. If exam is going smoothly, a goal of five good pieces of tissue is reasonable.
5. If lung collapse occurs, a chest tube may be inserted for lung re-expansion.

Potential Complications

1. Same as Flexible Bronchoscopy
2. Severe to moderate bleeding
3. Pneumothorax
4. Subcutaneous and mediastinal emphysema occurs rarely

Post Procedure Assessment/Care

1. Same as Flexible Bronchoscopy.
2. Alert the patient that he/she may cough up blood post biopsy.
3. If difficulty breathing and pain occurs, and is not relieved by patient's standard inhalation medications, the physician should be notified. If severe, 911 should be called.
4. Instruct the patient to avoid the ingestion of aspirin or aspirin-containing products, or non-steroidal anti-inflammatories for a period of time as per physician recommendations.

References

Bordow, R.A., Morris, T. A. & Ries, A.L. (2005). *Manual of Clinical Problems in Pulmonary Medicine* (6th ed.). Philadelphia: Lippincott, Williams & Wilkins.

Lesser, S. (2004). Bronchoscopy for the New Endoscopy Nurse. *Endonurse.* Virgo Publishing. Retrieved on 11/2/06 from http://www.endonurse.com/articles/2002/05/bronchoscopy-for-the-new-endoscopy-nurse.aspx.

Prakash, U.B.S., (1994) *Bronchoscopy* pp 122-128, 141-145, 369. New York: Raven Press.

Wang, K., Mebileu, A.C. Turner, F. (2004). *Flexible Bronchoscopy* (2nd ed.). Malden: Blackwell Publishing.

Bronchial Brushings

(Use in conjunction with Flexible Bronchoscopy, page 1)

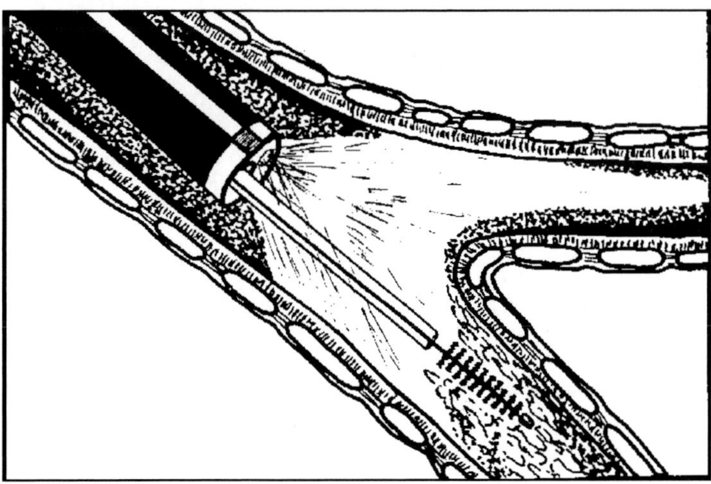

Figure 14: Endobronchial brushing

Description

Bronchial brushings uses a cytology brush to obtain samples of the respiratory mucosa under direct bronchoscopic or fluoroscopic guidance. By agitating the brush along the mucosa, a mixture of respiratory tract mucus that may contain infecting organisms and epithelial cells is obtained. The contents of the brush are analyzed for culture and/or cytology. Thus, the major uses of the brush are for diagnosis of lower respiratory infections (pneumonia) and for diagnosis of endobronchal lesions (lung cancer). The choice of brush type and technique vary with the underlying abnormality.

Indications

1. Endobronchial mass or obstruction
2. Pneumonia – ventilator associated
3. Pneumonia – unusual community acquired, e.g., Tuberculosis or immunocompromised patient

Contraindications

Contraindications describe circumstances in which a particular procedure is not usually performed. In some circumstances, however, the needs of the patient may require that a procedure proceed despite the presence of the condition. The physician makes these decisions.

1. Bleeding diathesis including coagulopathy and thrombocytopenia
2. Respiratory failure requiring high FIO_2 or PEEP

Pre-Procedure Assessment/Care

Same as Flexible Bronchoscopy.

Patient Teaching

1. Same as Flexible Bronchoscopy.
2. Reassure patient that brushing procedure is painless.

3. Inform patient of what may be heard during the process of brush biopsies (e.g., "brush out" and "brush in").
4. Reassure patient it is common to have some bleeding after brush biopsies are performed; however, coughing up more than two tablespoons of blood should be reported to the physician.
5. Inform patient when and how the results of the biopsies can be obtained.

Equipment

1. Sterile cytology brush of selected type
   a. Cytology brush consists of a wire with a rigid brush attached to the distal end. The wire with its brush tip is contained within a plastic sheath that is passed through the working channel of a flexible bronchoscope. When the wire is advanced, the brush tip extends beyond the protective sheath and can be directed to contact the airway.
   b. Protected brush (sometimes known as a microbiology brush) – brush is protected from the environment by a plug in the tip of the sheath which can be extruded within the lung at time of sampling.
2. Sterile glass slides
3. Cytology fixative (spray or alcohol fixative)
4. Non-bacteriostatic saline
5. Sterile scissors or wire cutters
6. Gauze sponges

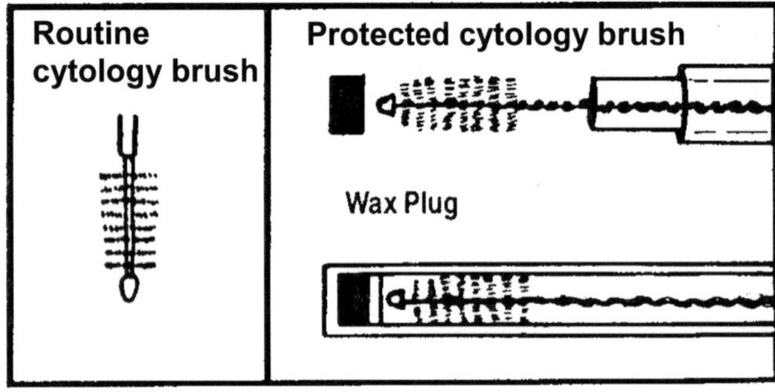

Figure 15: Cytology brushes

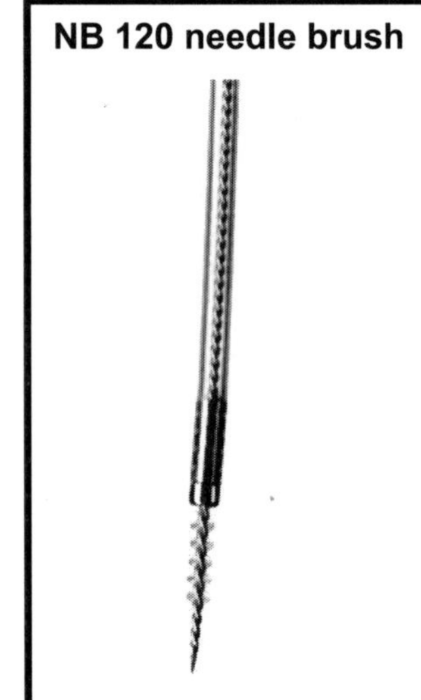

Figure 16: NB 120 needle brush [illustration courtesy of Bard Endoscopic Technologies]

Responsibilities During Procedure

1. Same as Flexible Bronchoscopy.
2. Properly handle and label all specimens.
3. Assist physician as the cytology brush is passed.
4. Advance and withdraw cytology brush at the physician's request. NOTE: The brush should only be advanced through the bronchoscope while within the protective sheath.
5. Withdraw the cytology brush from the channel in the closed position.
6. When withdrawing the brush, wipe the shaft with a gauze sponge to remove secretions.
7. Specimens are prepared and submitted following institutional policy and physician request.
   a. Specimens may be transferred to a glass slide by pressing the bristles of the brush against the slide. Cells should be transferred in a circular motion of the brush against the slide.

The specimen is then fixed onto the slide by spraying with cytology fixative spray or immersing slide into an alcohol fixative.

b. Brush may be agitated and/or cut off into a tube containing a small volume of sterile saline or other solution appropriate for the type of test to be performed.

Potential Complications

Same as Flexible Bronchoscopy.

Post-Procedure Assessment/Care

1. Same as Flexible Bronchoscopy.
2. If chest x-ray is ordered by physician to rule out pneumothorax, notify physician promptly of results.
3. Alert the patient that blood may be expectorated post procedure. If bleeding is persistent, the physician should be notified.

References

Ernst A, Editor. (2009). *Introduction to Bronchoscopy.* New York: Cambridge University Press.

Looi K, Sutanto EN, Banerjee B, Garratt L, Ling KM, Foo CJ, Stick SM, Kicic A. (2011). Bronchial brushings for investigating airway inflammation and remodelling. *Respirology,* 16, 725-737.

Prakash, U. B. (1994). *Bronchoscopy.* New York: Raven Press.

Wilkins, R. & Sheldon, R. (2005). *Clinical Assessment in Respiratory Care* (5th edition). Philadelphia: Mosby, Inc.

Bronchoalveolar Lavage/Washings

(Use in conjunction with Flexible Bronchoscopy, page 1, or Flexible Bronchoscopy (Pediatric), page 7)

Description

Bronchoalveolar lavage (BAL) is a commonly-used method of obtaining samples of material from the distal lung. It involves the "flooding" of a pulmonary subsegment (including distal airways and alveoli) with sterile non-bacteriostatic saline, followed by suctioning of the instilled fluid. (Note that only 40-60% of instilled fluid will probably be removed.) Lavage involves large amounts of fluid, as much as 300cc, while washing involves only a small amount (5 - 10cc). The lavage fluid can then be used in cytologic, microbiologic and chemical analysis.

Indications

1. Pneumonia
2. Interstitial lung disease
3. Alveolar hemorrhage
4. Alveolar proteinosis
5. Quantitative cultures for ventilator associated pneumonia

Contraindications

Contraindications describe circumstances in which a particular procedure is not usually performed. In some circumstances, however, the needs of the patient may require that a procedure proceed despite the presence of the condition. The physician makes these decisions.

1. Bleeding diathesis - severe thrombocytopenia or coagulopathy
2. Respiratory failure requiring high FIO_2 or PEEP
3. Cardiac instability
4. Uncooperative patient
5. Acute asthmatic episode (active bronchospasm)
6. Hypoxia, unless patient is intubated
7. NPO status not met

Patient Teaching

Same as Flexible Bronchoscopy

Pre-Procedure Assessment/Care

Same as Flexible Bronchoscopy

Equipment

1. Same as Flexible Bronchoscopy
2. In-line suction set up

Responsibilities During Procedure

1. Assist the physician with bronchoscopy procedure. The tip of the scope will be wedged into the subsegment to be lavaged. The lower and middle lobes are most often lavaged due to the higher rate of return of lavage fluid.
2. Assist the physician with instillation of normal saline into suction channel to cleanse the channel.
3. As the physician wedges the scope, the assistant instills aliquots of sterile non-bacteriostatic normal saline using a non-Luer-Lok syringe. *Especially for children and the elderly: smaller*

Specimen Collection

aliquots may be used for patients with special needs (particularly for pediatric and frail elderly patients.)

4. The specimen is withdrawn into an in-line trap or aspirated manually into a syringe
5. Specimens are prepared and submitted following institutional policy and procedure.
6. If lavaging from several sites in lung, specimens may be separated at the direction of the physician. Identify site of each specimen on label.
7. Document the volume of solution instilled and the volume returned.

Potential Complications

1. Same as Flexible Bronchoscopy
2. Pleurisy

Post-Procedure Assessment/Care

Same as Flexible Bronchoscopy

References

Ahmed, A., & Ahmed, S., (2004). Oct-Dec; Comparison of bronchoalveolar lavage and cytology and transbronchial biopsy in the diagnosis of carcinoma of the lung. *Journal of Ayub Medical College (JAMC),* 16(4), 29-33.

American Thoracic Society: Critical Care Medicine. Bronchoalveolar Lavage. Retrieved on Feb. 3, 2012 from http://www.thoracic.org/clinical/critical-care/critical-care-procedures/bronchoalveolar-lavage.php.

Ernst A. (Ed.). (2009). *Introduction to Bronchoscopy.* New York: Cambridge University Press.

Feinsilver, S.H. & Fein, A.M. (Eds). (1995). *Textbook of Bronchoscopy.* Baltimore: Williams & Wilkins.

Georage, R., Light, R., Matthay,M. & Matthay, R. (Eds). (2005). *Chest Medicine Essentials of Pulmonary and Critical Care Medicine,* Fifth edition. Philadelphia: Lippincott, Williams & Wilkins.

Hattotawa, K. et al. (2002). Safety of bronchoscopy, biopsy, and BAL in research of patients with COPD. *CHEST,* 122, 1909-1912.

Looi K, Sutanto EN, Banerjee B, Garratt L, Ling KM, Foo CJ, Stick SM, Kicic A. (2011). Bronchial brushings for investigating airway inflammation and remodelling. *Respirology,* 16, 725-737.

Path, P. (2003). Methods for the assessment of endobronchial biopsy in clinical research and the effects of treatment. *American Journal of Respiratory and Critical Care Medicine,* 168, S1-S17.

Prakash, U.B. (1994). *Bronchoscopy.* New York: Raven Press.

Torres, A., & El-Ebiary, M. (1998). Invasive diagnostic techniques for pneumonia: Protected specimen brush, bronchoalveolar lavage, and lung biopsy methods. *Infectious Disease Clinics of North America,* 12, 701-722.

Wang, K., & Mehta, A. C. (2012). *Flexible bronchoscopy* (3rd ed.). Cambridge, MA: Blackwell Science.

Transbronchial Needle Aspiration

(Use in conjunction with Flexible Bronchoscopy, page 1)

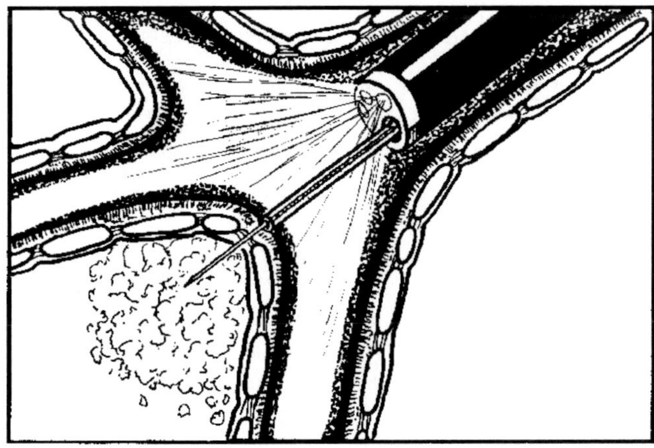

Figure 17: Transbronchial needle aspiration

Description

Transbronchial needle aspiration is the only technique that allows the bronchoscopist to sample tissue from beyond the confines of the endobronchial tree. Using an aspiration needle during bronchoscopy, cytology samples are obtained for microscopic examination.

Indications

1. Abnormal mass or nodes extrinsic to the bronchus
2. Abnormal radiologic studies with normal bronchoscopic examination
3. Staging of lymph nodes in known malignancy

Contraindications

Contraindications describe circumstances in which a particular procedure is not usually performed. In some circumstances, however, the needs of the patient may require that a procedure proceed despite the presence of the condition. The physician makes these decisions.

1. Same as Flexible Bronchoscopy.
2. Transbronchial needle biopsy not indicated when bacterial pneumonia is suspected.

Pre-Procedure Assessment/Care

Same as Flexible Bronchoscopy.

Patient Teaching

1. Same as Flexible Bronchoscopy.
2. Inform the patient that blood may be expectorated post biopsy.
3. Inform patient when and how the results of the biopsies can be obtained.

Equipment

NOTE: Fluoroscopy may be used. Endoscopic ultrasound may be used.

1. Same as Flexible Bronchoscopy
2. Transbronchial cytology needles of various sizes and shapes
3. Syringe (for aspiration)

4. On-site cytology for immediate diagnosis through tissue confirmation with operable microscope. If specimens are not prepared by Cytology staff immediately after they are obtained, have the following supplies available:
   a. glass slides
   b. slide fixative
   c. preservative
   d. non-bacteriostatic sterile normal saline or other solution required for the test ordered

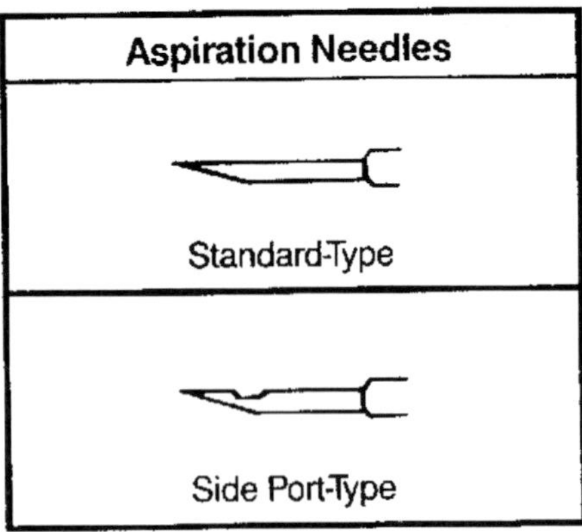

Figure 18: Aspiration needle types

Responsibilities During Procedure

1. Same as Flexible Bronchoscopy.
2. The physician advances the aspiration needle through the bronchoscope tip while it is in a straight position. To avoid damage to the biopsy channel, the bronchoscope is flexed only after the needle is extended beyond the tip of the scope into the visual field.
3. Remove obturator and stylet, if applicable.
4. Attach a syringe to the needle catheter (may prefer Luer-Lok connection to ensure tight seal).
5. The physician will advance and agitate the transbronchial needle while the assistant is applying vacuum with the syringe to obtain the specimen.
6. Pull needle back into sheath and withdraw from bronchoscope.
7. Immediately alert physician if blood is noted in syringe during aspiration.
8. Inject specimen into container (or onto slides).
9. Specimens are prepared and submitted according to institutional policy.

Potential Complications

1. Same as Flexible Bronchoscopy
2. Air embolus
3. Pneumomediastinum

Post Procedure Assessment/Care

1. Same as Flexible Bronchoscopy
2. Observe for respiratory distress (subcutaneous emphysema and tracheal deviation)
3. Alert the patient that blood may be expectorated post biopsy. If bleeding is persistent, the physician should be notified.

References

Bilaceroghu, S., et al. (2004). Transbronchial Needle Aspiration in Diagnosis of Intrathoracic Lymphadenitis. *CHEST*, 126, 259-267.

Bordow, R.A., Morris, T. A. & Ries, A.L. (2005). *Manual of Clinical Problems in Pulmonary Medicine* (6th ed.). Philadelphia: Lippincott, Williams & Wilkins.

Chokhani, R. (2004). Transbronchial needle aspiration in the diagnosis of respiratory diseases. *Nepal Med Coll. J*, 6(1), 24-7.

Feinsilver, S.H., & Fein, A.M. (Eds). (1995). *Textbook of bronchoscopy* . Baltimore: Williams & Wilkins.

Herth, R. Becker, H., Ernst, A. (2004). Conventional vs endobronchial ultrasound-guided transbronchial needle aspiration. *CHEST,* 125, 322-325.

Iglesias, J., Dominguez-Munoz, J. E., Abdulkader, I., Larino-Noia, J., Eugenyeva, E., Lozano-Leon, A., Forteza-Vila, J. (2011). Influence of on-site cytopathology evaluation on the diagnostic accuracy of endoscopic ultrasound-guided fine needle aspirations (EUS-FNA) of solid pancreatic masses. *The American Journal of Gastroenterology*, 106, 1705-1710.

Jinwoo, L, Young S. P., Seok-Chung, Y. (2011) The endoscopic cryotherapy of lung and bronchila tumors: A systemic review- can we expect a new era of cryotherapy in lung cancer? *The Korean Journal of Internal Medicine*, 26*(2),* 132-134.

Karan, N., Tuksavul, Edipoglu, O., Ermete, S., Guelu, S.Z. (2005). Effectiveness of transbronchial needle aspiration in the diagnosis of exophytic endobronchial lesions and submucosa/peribronchial disease of the lung. *Lung Cancer,* 50(2), 221-226.

Mason, R., Broaddus, V., Murray, J., & Nadel, J. (Eds). (2005). *Textbook of Respiratory Medicine* (4th ed.), (vol. 1). Philadelphia: W.B. Saunders.

Medford, A., R. L., Bennett, J., A., Free, C. M., Argrawal, S. (2010). Endobronchial ultrasound guided transbronchial needle aspiration. *Postgrad Medical Journal,* 86, 106-115.

Oki, M, Salka, H. Kumazawa, A., Sako, C., Ando, M., Watanube, A., (2004). The role of the transcarinal needle aspiration in the diagnosis and staging of lung cancer: computed tomographic correlation of a positive result. *RESPIRATION,* 71(5), 523-527.

Wang, K.R. et al. (2012). *Flexible Bronchoscopy* (3rd ed.*).* Cambridge, MA: Blackwell Science.

Win, T., et al. (2003). The role of transbronchial needle aspiration in the diagnosis of bronchogenic carcinoma. *Respiratory Care*, 48(6), 602-605.

Yasfuku, K., et al. (2004) Real-time endobronchial ultrasound guided transbronchial needle aspiration of mediastinal and hilar lymph nodes. *CHEST*, 126, 122-128.

Part 4

SAFETY

Safety

Description

It is the legal, ethical and moral responsibility of all endoscopy or bronchoscopy personnel to be aware of these safety standards and how they affect patient care. The following conditions and directions are general guidelines for maintaining safety. Blood and body fluid precautions and Standard Precautions are practiced for each patient. Occupational Safety and Health Administration (OSHA) and institutional policies and guidelines should be followed.

Environmental Safety

1. Use appropriate precautions with flammable gases or liquids.
2. Keep hallways and doorways free of equipment and carts.
3. Keep rooms neat and orderly.
4. Electrical cords, cable and tubing should be placed so personnel do not trip and fall.
5. All rooms must be adequately ventilated.
6. Ensure compliance with OSHA standards.
7. Conduct periodic evaluations for ergonomic considerations of repetitive movements. e.g., >2 hours of manually cleaning bronchoscopes using the same repetitive movements.
8. When occupied, patient stretchers, pre-and post-procedure, should be maintained in low position relative to the floor with side rails up to prevent falls.
9. Unoccupied patient stretchers should have brakes engaged at all times to minimize potential falls. *Especially for Children: Provide constant observation of children, and ensure that chemicals and equipment are kept out of their reach.*

Infection Control

1. Initiate TB algorithm at first contact with patients for early detection of tuberculosis.
2. Provide puncture-resistant containers to transport biohazardous materials, including endoscopes.
3. Plan preventive maintenance for all automated reprocessors.
4. Use Personal Protective Equipment whenever there is a possibility of splash of contaminated blood or body fluids.
    a. impervious gown with cuffed sleeves
    b. face shield to protect mouth, eyes, nose (all mucus membranes) or goggles and face mask
    c. gloves
    d. gloves that extend beyond cuffed sleeves of gown when decontaminating equipment

Chemical Safety

1. Read and follow label directions for all products for precautions, time, temperature, dilution for optimum performance.
2. Clearly identify liquid chemical germicides/sterilants (e.g., glutaraldehyde, peracetic acid) as biohazardous.
3. Monitor vapor per OSHA guidelines: initially, annually and at any signs or symptoms of overexposure.
4. Ensure appropriate vapor containment: tightly covered containers, fume hoods, etc.
5. Keep MSDS sheets readily accessible.
6. Use absorptive products to help absorb vapors.
7. Provide spill containment plans for the chemicals you use; keep neutralizing agents readily available.

8. Use personal protective equipment, including polyethylene, butyl rubber or nitrile rubber gloves at least 11″ long that overlap cuffed sleeves of impervious gown.
9. Have available a hands-free, cold water only, eyewash station for emergency use in each area where chemical products are used.
10. Ensure room ventilation that meets national standards in areas where liquid chemical germicides/sterilants are used (10 air exchanges per hour).
11. Provide annual inservices on safe use of liquid chemical germicides/sterilants.

Electrical Safety

1. Maintain electrical cords in safe working order.
2. Ascertain that all electrical equipment is property grounded.
3. Do not use multiple-outlet adapters or two-wire extension cords.
4. Do not remove ground pins from three-pin plugs.
5. Avoid routing power lines through heavy traffic areas.
6. Follow manufacturer's recommendations and standards for all equipment.
7. Report and have repaired any malfunctioning equipment or potential hazard immediately.
8. Inspect all cables frequently for breaks or frays.
9. Report all malfunctioning equipment immediately and take appropriate action.
10. Always use lowest acceptable power settings, confirmed verbally to the endoscopist before activation.
11. Perform and document periodic checks on all electrical equipment.
12. Because liquids are excellent conductors of electricity, never place a container of liquid on or near electrical equipment.
13. Never use light source as a supply table. Essential equipment must be plugged into a red outlet to ensure continuous electrical supply.

Electrocautery Safety

1. Place dispersive electrode (formerly called grounding pad) properly on the patient: muscular, well vascularized site, away from bony prominences, scar tissue or where circulation is likely to be impaired, metal plates, pins or joints.
2. Avoid current flow close to the site of a cardiac pacemaker.
3. Patients with implanted cardiac defibrillating device should have the device inactivated by a trained practitioner/cardiologist before undergoing procedure where there is a likelihood of electrosurgery device use.
4. Test equipment prior to procedure per manufacturer's instructions.
5. **When argon is being used, it is essential that the nurse or associate visually and verbally verify that supplemental oxygen is turned off prior to and during each firing of the APC probe if the oxygen level being used is 40% or more. If the oxygen is 40% or less, the oxygen does not need to be completely turned off.**

Latex Precautions

1. Reduce exposure and risk for development of latex allergy.
2. Use powder-free gloves if latex gloves are chosen for protection from blood or body fluids.
3. Avoid latex-containing products, e.g., gloves, balloons, dilators, to avoid sensitization and possible occupation-induced asthma.
4. Provide education about latex allergy.
5. Assess patient's predisposition or actual allergy to latex.
6. Identify individuals in the high-risk group for latex sensitization or allergy.
7. If a patient has a latex allergy, clearly post an allergy alert, easily visible to all personnel around the patient and follow institutional policy for dealing with a patient who is allergic to

latex. Make every effort to have patients with latex allergies scheduled as first procedure of the day.

8. Check manufacturer's information to verify that band ligators, dilators, etc. are latex-free.

Equipment Safety

1. Perform and document inspection of all equipment on an established schedule.
2. Pre-procedure bronchoscope checks should include the following
   a. Turn on light source and suction to make sure both are functioning properly.
   b. Check air/water channel.
   c. Look through scope or check video image for broken fiber bundles, presence of fluid or poor visualization.
   d. Test bronchoscopes for leakage after each use.
   e. Check for bite marks or indication of damage on scope.
   f. Manipulate all controls.
3. Electrocautery precautions:
   a. Test equipment prior to procedure per manufacturer's instructions.
   b. Ground patient and equipment per manufacturer's instructions.

Laser Safety

1. Place a warning sign on the door leading into the room where laser is in use.
2. Provide protective eyewear for patients and personnel that provide proper optical density.
3. Use instruments that are anodized or that have a non-reflective coating.
4. Keep laser in standby mode; allow only one hand set accessibility by physician when in use.
5. Use lasers with tamper-proof audio tones.
6. Use smoke evacuators and high-filtration masks to minimize smoke inhalation, when applicable.
7. Do not use flammable or combustible materials near the laser site.
8. Use inline filter for scope suction.

Radiation Safety

1. Inservices regarding radiation safety should be conducted for personnel on an annual basis.
2. X-ray badges (dosimeters) should be worn by all personnel during procedures when radiation exposure is encountered, at the thyroid area and under lead apron at the pocket level.
3. Analyze exposure levels monthly.
4. Wear lead aprons and thyroid collars and observe other proper shielding precautions as per institution guidelines.
5. Use leaded glasses for personnel closest to the patient.
6. Use a lead curtain around the fluoroscopy tower, if available.
7. Pregnant personnel should not regularly assist with x-ray procedures. If a staff member is pregnant, contact your institution's radiation safety officer for recommendations on additional safety measures to be taken for fetal safety.
8. All female patients of childbearing age should be questioned about the possibility of pregnancy before x-ray procedure. If patient is of childbearing age, shield patient's pelvis.
9. While fluoroscope is in use, personnel should not turn unshielded backs to x-ray unit and should maintain as great a distance as possible.
10. Institutional policies regarding x-ray exposure should be known and followed by personnel participating in x-ray procedures.
11. Check lead aprons regularly to ensure they meet standards of protection from radiation.

Post-Sedation Safety

1. Monitor vital signs per institution guidelines.
2. If local anesthesia is applied to the throat, keep patient NPO until gag reflex returns.
3. Keep side rails elevated.
4. Assist patient with ambulation as needed.
5. Provide continuous observation for sedated patients.
6. Instruct outpatients who have received sedation not to drive, operate heavy machinery or drink alcohol for a period of time which is appropriate for the medications given (see drug manufacturer's guidelines or drug information source).
7. Provide post-procedure written instructions for outpatients and provide verbal report to nurse responsible for inpatient's care.
8. Follow all other institution guidelines for the sedated patient.

Patient Emergency Situation Safety

1. Follow institution policies for fire, severe weather and other disasters.
2. Bronchoscopy unit should be equipped with the following:
   a. oxygen
   b. crash cart with appropriate equipment and medications
   c. chest-tube set-up with various size tubes
   d. CPR trained personnel; personnel trained in Advanced Life Support immediately available.
   e. personnel knowledgeable in the use of medications, recognizing side effects and types of antagonists to be used

   Especially for Children

   All medical facilities involved in the care of children must be prepared for the possibility of a life-threatening emergency. Personnel trained in advanced life support techniques (pediatric and neonatal, if applicable) must be immediately available should an emergency arise. The pediatric emergency "crash" cart should be stocked with equipment in a variety of sizes appropriate for the age groups receiving care in the facility.

   Nurses involved in the sedation and monitoring of children who undergo diagnostic and therapeutic procedures should be aware of age-related normal values for vital signs, and should be prepared to act quickly in the event of vital sign changes which suggest a possible complication. Dosages of sedative medications to be given (in mg per kg) may vary between institutions, ordering physician and according to patient need. However, nurses who administer sedative medications to children need to have a thorough knowledge of recommended dosages, as well as appropriate monitoring protocols and use of antagonists, if needed.

References

Acello, B. (2002). *The OSHA Handbook: The Guidelines for Compliance In Health* (3rd ed.). Florence, KY: Thomson Delmar Learning.

Chobin, N. (1999). Recommended good practices for cleaning and disinfection. *Infection Control and Sterilization Technology,* 5, 41-44.

Feigenbaum, K. , Ellet, M.L., Miller, R., & Hyland, L. (1998). ALARA study of teaching effectiveness on reducing radiation exposure. *Gastroenterology Nursing,* 21, 234-238.

Gannon, P.F., Bright, P., Campbell, M., O"Hickey, S.P., & Burge, P.S., (1995). Occupational asthma due to glutaraldehyde and formaldehyde in endoscopy and X-ray departments. *Thorax*, 50, 156-159.

Lechtman, M.D. (1999) Understanding disinfectants and antiseptic labeling, with some emphasis on testing. *Infection Control and Sterilization Technology,* 5, 28-32.

Rayhorn, N. (1998). Sedating and monitoring pediatric patients: Defining the nurse's responsibilities from preparation through recovery. *American Journal of Maternal/Child Nursing,* 23, 76-86.

Roberts, E. (Ed.). (2005). *Infection Control in Respiratory Care: Strategies for JCAHO Compliance.* Marblehead, MA: HCPro, Inc.

Rutala, W.A., Weber, D.J. (2001). *New Disinfection and Sterilization Methods.* CDC, 7(2).

Rutala, W.A. (Ed). (1998). *Disinfection, sterilization and antisepsis in healthcare.* Washington DC: Association for Professionals in Infection Control and Epidemiology, Inc.

Society of Gastroenterology Nurses and Associates, Inc. (2009) *Endoscope cleaning and high level disinfection* (4th ed.) (video study module). Chicago: Author.

Society of Gastroenterology Nurses and Associates, Inc. (SGNA). (2010) *Guidelines for Preventing Reactions to Natiural Rubber Latex in the Workplace* [Guideline]. Chicago: Author.

Society of Gastroenterology Nurses and Associates, Inc. (SGNA). (2008) *Radiation Safety in the Endoscopy Setting* [Guideline]. Chicago: Author.

Society of Gastroenterology Nurses and Associates, Inc. (SGNA). (2007). *Guidelines for the use of high-level disinfectants and sterilants for reprocessing of flexible gastrointestinal endoscopes* [Guideline]. Chicago: Author.

Society of Gastroenterology Nurses and Associates, Inc. (SGNA). (2009). *Standard of Infection Control in Reprocessing of Flexible gastrointestinal endoscopes* [Guideline]. Chicago: Author.

Society of Gastroenterology Nurses and Associates, Inc. (SGNA). (2009). *Standards of clinical nursing practice* and role delineations [Guideline]. Chicago: Author.

Part 5

STANDARD EQUIPMENT FOR PULMONARY ENDOSCOPIC PROCEDURES

STANDARD EQUIPMENT FOR PULMONARY ENDOSCOPIC PROCEDURES

Description

Standard equipment and supplies are needed for every endoscopic procedure. Equipment is checked prior to the start of all procedures. The manufacturer's instructions are followed for cleaning, disinfecting and/or sterilizing all equipment. Personnel maintain accurate knowledge of equipment functioning, handling and maintenance.

Equipment

1. Endoscope of choice
2. Light source/video system
3. Two suction sources (one for mouth, one for scope)
4. Electrocautery equipment and grounding pads
5. Blood pressure cuffs of various sizes and stethoscope or blood pressure monitor
6. Supplemental oxygen and oxygen delivery system (nasal cannula/mask/trach collar)
7. EKG monitor available
8. Pulse oximeter
9. Teaching attachment (optional)
10. Equipment for cardiopulmonary emergency (crash cart)
11. Chest tube set-up

NOTE: Non-latex alternatives must be available for use by sensitive and allergic patients and personnel.

Accessory Supplies

1. Biopsy forceps
2. Snares
3. Retrieval forceps
4. Cytology brushes
5. Cytology containers with preservative
6. Histology/pathology containers with preservative
7. Labels for specimen labeling
8. Sterile containers
9. Non-bacteriostatic saline
10. Sterile suction trap container
11. Laboratory specimen slips
12. Irrigation supplies
13. Electrosurgical accessories
14. Laser probes
15. Magnetic extractors
16. Balloon catheters
17. Lukens trap
18. Sterile gauze and ampules of sterile saline for possible fresh section/biopsy
19. Injection therapy needle and saline or epinephrine solution for potential bleeding

Miscellaneous Supplies

1. Syringes and needles
2. Personal protective equipment
3. Gauze sponges

4. Silicone
5. Local anesthetics
6. Medications for sedation
7. Drug reversal agents
8. Camera, film, video tape
9. Suction tubing and catheters/oral suction device
10. Mouthpiece/bite block
11. IV solutions and IV tubing, IV pole
12. IV catheters in various sizes and lengths
13. Non-latex glove assortment

Additional Equipment and Supplies for Pediatrics

1. Calculator for checking dosages and amounts of medications
2. Tuberculin syringes to ensure accuracy of measurement
3. Pediatric size oximeter probes
4. Blood pressure cuffs in varied sizes; same size for entire stay
5. Pediatric emergency cart
6. Accurate weight in kilograms
7. Immobilization device (Papoose Board)
8. Endoscope accessories (biopsy forceps, graspers, etc.) which are compatible with the size of the instrument being used.
9. IV cannulae in a variety of sizes commonly used for children (i.e., 27, 24, 22g)
10. Microdrip IV tubing and buretrol for controlled fluid delivery
11. Endotracheal tubes

Reference

Shankar, V., Deshpancle. (2005). Sedation for the pediatric patient – a review. *Pediatric Clinics of North America,* 23(4), 635-654.

Society of Gastroenterology Nurses and Associates. (2008). *Gastroenterology Nursing: A core curriculum.* (4th ed.). Chicago: Author.

APPENDICES

Appendix A

Medications Commonly Used During Pulmonary Procedures

The medications listed here are representative of frequently-used drugs at specific sites. Please keep in mind that your site and practitioner may use different medications, or the same medications at different dosages. This section is designed to be a point of reference and not an all-inclusive medication list for pulmonary procedures.

The tables following highlight specific information for each drug.

Indications	Dose & Route	Contraindications	Responsibilities During Administration	Potential Complications
Acetylcysteine (Mucomyst)				
• Presence of thick secretions in the respiratory tract that make breathing difficult • Decreases mucus viscosity, allowing mobilization and expectoration	• Nebulization via facemask • Mouthpiece or tracheotomy or directly via bronchoscope **Adult** • 1-10 ml of 20% solution, or 2 – 20 ml of 10% solution q 2-6 hours **Pediatric** • 3-5 ml of 20% solution (diluted with equal volume of water or sterile saline to equal 10%) –or- • 6-10 ml of 10% solution	• Status asthmaticus • Pregnancy • Nursing mother • Decreased ability to cough • Hypersensitivity	• Explain to patient the need to deep breathe and cough before treatment • Advise patient medication smells like rotten eggs • Suction through bronchoscope and oral cavity PRN	• Expectorating blood in mucus • Hemoptysis • Bronchospasm • Angioedema • Anaphylaxis • Wheezing • Chest tightness • Difficulty breathing • Increased secretions • Nausea and vomiting • Drowsiness • Rhinorrhea

Indications	Dose & Route	Contraindications	Responsibilities During Administration	Potential Complications
Albuterol Sulfate Inhalation Solution (Ventolin or Proventil)				
• Bronchodilator • Prevention or relief of bronchospasm	• Nebulization via facemask • Unit dose is equivalent to 2.5 mg albuterol sulfate in 3 ml normal saline **<u>Adult</u>** • Adjust flow rate of nebulizer to deliver 2.5 mg albuterol over 5-15 minutes **<u>Pediatric</u>** <u>Neonate-infant</u> • 0.05 – 0.15 mg/kg/dose <u>1-5 years</u> • 2.5 mg/dose <u>over 12 years</u> • 2.5-5mg/dose	• Tachycardia • Severe cardiac disease • Heart block • Hypersensitivity • Pregnancy (relative) • Nursing mothers (relative)	• Protect medication from light until ready to use • Do not use if markedly discolored • Administer medication slowly • Ensure proper use of nebulizer • Unit dose must be used immediately and any un-used portion discarded appropriately • Do not expose to temperatures over 86 degrees	• Paradoxical bronchospasm • Tremors • Anxiety • Insomnia • Headache • Palpitations • Tachycardia • Deterioration of asthma

Indications	Dose & Route	Contraindications	Responsibilities During Administration	Potential Complications
Atropine Sulfate				
• Decrease oral and respiratory secretions • Increase bronchodilation • Inhibit vasovagal reaction	**Adult** • 0.0 to 1.0 mg IV, immediately prior to giving moderate sedation **Pediatric** • 0.01 mg/kg/dose • Maximum dose 0.4mg • Minimum dose 0.1 mg	• Paralytic Ileus • Closed angle glaucoma • Acute hemorrhage • Tachycardia secondary to cardiac insufficiency and thyrotoxicosis • Known allergy • Ulcerative colitis or toxic megacolon • Severe renal disease • Myasthenia gravis • Severe hepatic disease	• Continuous cardiac monitoring; notify physician of changes in HR, BP or ventricular ectopy • Explain to patient that increased heart rate is normal and expected • Use glycerin swabs to relieve dry mouth post-procedure • Promptly report significant changes in HR, BP, or increased ventricular ectopy to physician	• Tachycardia • Coma • Urinary retention/ hesitancy • Constipation • Drowsiness • Blurred vision • Impaired ability to judge distance • Confusion • Dry mouth • Palpitations • Blurred vision

Indications	Dose & Route	Contraindications	Responsibilities During Administration	Potential Complications
Codeine Sulfate				
• Decrease response to pain • Suppress cough mechanism	• Given post-procedure **Adult** • PO 15-60 mg q 4-6 h (usual adult dose is 30mg) • Not to exceed 120 mg/day **Pediatric** 1 year or older: 0.5 mg/kg body weight every 4 to 6 hours 2-6 years • 2.5-5 mg/dose q 4-6 h 6-12 years • 5-10 mg/dose q 4-6 h	• Respiratory depression • MAO inhibitors within 14 days (Parenate, Marplan, Nardil & Eatron) • Pregnancy • Nursing mothers • Frequent ingestion of alcohol • Use of Tagamet (cimetadine) • Bronchial asthma • Raised intracranial pressure • <2 years of age	• Reduce dosage if liver impairment • Reduce dosage if renal insufficiency • Do not use if solution is discolored or if there is precipitate • Mix with sterile water and filter when administering	• Respiratory paralysis • Anaphylaxis • Circulatory collapse • Seizures • Agitation/confusion • Lethargy/stupor • Urinary retention • Palpitations • Bradycardia
Diazepam (Valium)				
• Short-term relief of anxiety • Diminish patient recall of procedure	**Adult** • Initial dose: • 2.5 – 5 mg IV q 15 min • Up to 20 mg IV 30 minutes pre-procedure **Pediatric** • 0.25mg/kg/dose • Give slowly over 3 minutes; wait 15 to 20 minutes to administer 2nd dose. After additional 15-30 min may administer 3rd and last dose	• Closed angle glaucoma • Open angle glaucoma unless receiving appropriate therapy • Pregnancy, esp. 1st trimester • Myasthenia gravis • <6 mos. of age • Use with caution in debilitated patient, or patient with renal or hepatic disease • Sleep apnea	• Administer medication slowly – 5mg.min max • Have reversal drug available: Flumazenil (Romazicon) • Adheres to plastic IV tubing; be sure to flush well and use closest IV port to administer; administer via large veins	• Respiratory depression • Tachycardia • Neutropenia • Increased cough reflex • Laryngospasm • Hypotension • Venous thrombosis, phlebitis • Apnea • Cardiac arrest • Somnolence • Confusion • Coma

Indications	Dose & Route	Contraindications	Responsibilities During Administration	Potential Complications
Diphenhydramine (Benadryl)				
• Symptomatic relief of allergic reaction • Antihistamine and anticholinergic effect of drying secretions and mild sedation to enhance other medications used	**Adult** May be given undiluted by direct IV, 10-50 mg q 2-3 hours PRN • May need up to 100 mg dose • Not to exceed 300 mg/day **Pediatric** • 5 mg/kg/24 h divided q 6 h	• Lower respiratory disease such as an acute asthma attack • MAO inhibitors within previous 2 weeks • Narrow angle glaucoma • Pregnant or planning to become pregnant soon • Nursing mothers • Premature infant or neonate	• Do not use drug if discolored or has precipitate • Administer slowly, not to exceed 25 mg/min • Use caution when giving to patient with: - bronchial asthma - increased intraocular pressure - hyperthyroidism - hypertension - cardiac/renal disease	• Seizures • Anaphylaxis • Hallucinations • Sudden death • Hypotension • Palpitations • Tachycardia • Confusion/restlessness • Tightness in the chest or throat/wheezing • Photosensitivity may occur
Epinephrine 1:1000 (Adrenalin Chloride)				
• Nasal congestion • Superficial bleeding in the airways • Bronchodilator	**Adult** • Mix epinephrine (1:1000) with 9 cc of normal saline to equal epinephrine 1:10,000) • Instill 1-2 cc via bronchoscope **Pediatric** • 0.01 mg/kg/dose sq	• Closed angle glaucoma • Use with MAO inhibitors may lead to hypertensive crisis	• Assess face, lips or eyelids for swelling. If occurs, notify physician immediately. • Assess ECG continuously	• Paradoxical bronchospasm/wheeze • Dysrhythmias • Fatal ventricular fibrillation • Hypertension • Stroke • Cerebral hemorrhage • Restlessness/confusion • Tremors • Weakness • Dizziness • Sweating • Palpitations

Indications	Dose & Route	Contraindications	Responsibilities During Administration	Potential Complications
Fentanyl Citrate (Sublimaze)				
• Narcotic analgesic (relieves pain) • Suppress cough mechanism • Reduce anxiety • Reduce motor activity	**Adult** • 0.5-1 mcg/kg/dose • 25 – 50 mcg IV given in intermittent doses • Reduce doses in elderly • NOTE: Rapid IV infusion increases the incidence of serious side effects **Pediatric (over 2 years old)** • 1-2 mcg/kg/dose q 30-60 min	• Narrow angle glaucoma • Bone marrow depression • CNS depression • Severe liver/respiratory disease • Hypersensitivity to opiates • Myasthenia gravis • Breast feeding mothers • Pregnancy	• Have reversal drug available – Naloxone HCL (Narcan) • Administer medication slowly	• Respiratory depression/apnea • Cardiac arrest • Laryngospasm • Bradycardia • Increased cough • Hypotension or hypertension • Apnea • Somnolence • Confusion • Coma • Muscular rigidity
Flumazenil (Romazicon)				
• Smooth awakening from benzodiazepine-induced conscious sedation • Suspected benzodiazepine overdose	**Adult** • Initial dose: 0.2 mg (2 ml) IV over 15 seconds • If desired level of consciousness is not obtained after waiting an additional 45 seconds, give follow-up dose • Follow-up dose: additional 0.2 mg (2 ml) IV every 60 seconds to a maximum dose of 1 mg (10 ml) **Pediatric** • 2-3 mcg/kg IV	• Use care in patients with seizure history • Serious cyclic antidepressant overdose • Use cautiously in patients with long-term benzodiazepine use • Pregnancy (relative) • Nursing mothers • MAO inhibitors within 14 days	• Monitor level of consciousness, respirations, O_2 saturation • Be aware that re-sedation may occur within 2 hours	• Seizures • Dysrhythmias • Nausea • Vomiting • Headache • Agitation

Indications	Dose & Route	Contraindications	Responsibilities During Administration	Potential Complications
Lidocaine HCL 1% and 2% injection (Xylocaine)				
• Local or regional anesthesia by infiltration techniques such as percutaneous injection and intravenous regional anesthesia by peripheral nerve block techniques	• Route of administration determines dose	• Sensitivity to lidocaine • Breastfeeding mothers • Pregnancy	• Advise patient a mild, transient stinging sensation may occur after application	• Seizures • Heart block • Tremors • Twitching • Confusion • Convulsions • Bleeding
Lidocaine HCL 4% solution (Xylocaine)				
• Anesthetize the nose and upper airways	• 5cc (200 mg) of 40 mg/ml concentration via nebulizer approximately 20 minutes prior to bronchoscopy	• Severe Heart block • Blood dyscrasias • Sensitivity to lidocaine	• Have methylene blue available	• Seizures • Heart block • Methemoglobinemia • Vomiting • Hypotension collapse • Rash • Blurred vision
Lidocaine, 2% Viscous (Xylocaine)				
• Topical anesthesia of mucus membranes of the nose, mouth and pharynx • Suppress gag reflex during endoscopy or intubation	• Use smaller doses in the elderly or debilitated to decrease risk of toxicity	• Active, untreated infection of affected area • Do not use in the eye • Sensitivity to lidocaine	• Have methylene blue available	• Seizures • Hypotension/Cardiovascular collapse • Heart block • Methemoglobinemia • Respiratory depression • Vomiting • Rash • Blurred vision • Burning, stinging, tenderness, irritation

Indications	Dose & Route	Contraindications	Responsibilities During Administration	Potential Complications
Meperidine HCL (Demerol)				
• Narcotic analgesic • Suppress cough mechanism • Reduce anxiety	**Adult** • 25 – 50 mg IV in intermittent doses • NOTE: A rapid IV infusion increases the incidence of serious side effects • Reduce dose by half if currently taking phenothiazines **Pediatric** • 1-1.5 mg/kg/dose • Maximum dose = 100 mg • 1mg/kg to max of 3mg/kg	• MAO inhibitors within previous 2 weeks • Acute abdomen • Pregnancy except during labor • Nursing mothers • Renal failure (active metabolite may cause CNS irritability – seizures) • Sensitivity to Demerol • Patients with head injury	• Use with care if atrial fibrillation or other supraventricular tachycardias • Use caution in patients with impaired hepatic or renal function, hyper-thyroidism, Addison's disease, other debilitated patients; asthma; COPD; prostatic hypertrophy • Encourage patient to remain quiet and slightly reclining, if possible • Administer slowly • Have reversal agent (Narcan) readily accessible • May cause orthostatic hypotension	• Cardiac arrest • Respiratory depression • Increased intracranial pressure • Seizures • Anaphylaxis • Hypotension • Hallucinations and disorientation • Phlebitis at IV site

Indications	Dose & Route	Contraindications	Responsibilities During Administration	Potential Complications
Methylene Blue				
• Acts as electron donor to increase methemoglobin reduction • Reduces methemoglobin level by 50% within one hour	**Adult** • IV 1-2 mg/kg in a 1% solution slowly over 5 minutes followed by 10-15 cc saline flush • May repeat in 1 hr and every 4 hr **Pediatric** • 1-2 mg/kg	• Not effective for G6PD deficiency • Pregnancy • Breast feeding • Renal impairment • Hypersensitivity	• Realize that administration temporarily interferes with pulse oximetry readings • Wear gloves – will discolor skin	• Side effects: blue-green urine, GI distress (nausea & vomiting), hypertension, blue skin color • Acute hemolysis (if G6PD deficient) • Precordial pain, dyspnea, restlessness/confusion, hemolytic anemia, dysuria, diaphoresis (toxic) • Over-treatment may result in paradoxical formation of methemoglobin

Indications	Dose & Route	Contraindications	Responsibilities During Administration	Potential Complications
Methylprednisolone (Solu-Medrol)				
• Anti-inflammatory medication for asthmatic patients • Treatment of allergic reaction response • Adjunct for fulminating or disseminating pulmonary tuberculosis • Treatment for aspiration pneumonitis	**Adult** • 40-80 mg/day in 1-2 titratable doses **Pediatric** • 2 mg/kg/24 h divided q 6 h	• Women of childbearing age • Pregnant women • Nursing mothers • Premature infants • Systemic fungal infection • Tuberculosis • Psychosis	• Prepare for administration by mixing the powder medication with the provided diluent • Administer slowly over several minutes • Observe carefully and use caution for patients with: - hypothyroidism - cirrhosis - concurrent cyclosporin use	• Seizures • Hypertension • Cardiac dysrhythmias • Bronchospasm • Circulatory collapse • Bradycardia • Cardiac arrest • Hypotension • Patient to avoid exposure to chicken pox or measles • Psychotic changes

Indications	Dose & Route	Contraindications	Responsibilities During Administration	Potential Complications
Midazolam (Versed)				
• Sedation for diagnostic endoscopic procedures • Induces amnesia • Anxiety	**Adult** • Individualized dosage, increase with caution • Initially 0.5 mg IV; give additional 0.5 mg dose PRN up to a total dose of 2.5 mg over at least 2 minutes until desired effect is achieved • If additional necessary, wait 2 minutes after last dose, then give doses in 0.5 mg increments. • Total dose > 5 mg is rarely necessary **Pediatric** • 0.1 to 0.5mg/kg IV or IM initially • 6 months to 5 years – 0.6mg/kg IV • 6 to 12 years – 6 mg total • 1-2.5 mg IV over 2 min • Adjust to lowest effective dose	• Closed narrow angle glaucoma • Coma • Hypersensitivity to benzodiazepines • Congestive heart failure • Myasthenia gravis • Chronic renal failure(relative) • Intrathecal and epidural use • Status asthmaticus	• Have reversal drug available – Flumazenil (Romazicon) • Administer medication slowly • Have resuscitation equipment available	• Respiratory depression • Laryngospasm • Apnea • Bronchospasm • Circulatory depression • Respiratory arrest • Shock • Cardiac arrest • Hallucinations and disorientation • Phlebitis at intravenous site

Indications	Dose & Route	Contraindications	Responsibilities During Administration	Potential Complications
Naloxone HCL (Narcan)				
• Respiratory depression induced by narcotics • Antidote for opiate toxicity	**<u>Adult</u>** • Initially 0.4 – 2 mg IV over 15 seconds • May be repeated q 2-3 min up to a maximum of 10 mg • The duration of the opiate is often greater than that of naloxone; additional doses or continuous IV infusion might be necessary **<u>Pediatric</u>** <u>Neonates, infants and children < 20 kg</u> • 0.01 mg/kg/dose • may repeat q 2-3 minutes • Titrate to lowest effective response.	• Sensitivity to naloxone HCL	• Monitor ECG continuously • Caution: withdrawal in drug-dependent individuals may occur up to 2 hours after administration • Watch for re-sedation • Cautious use with patient with pre-existing cardiac disease	• Tachycardia/fibrillation • Pulmonary edema • Cardiac arrest • Seizures • Respiratory depression • Signs and symptoms of drug withdrawal in drug dependent individuals • Hypotension/hypertension

Indications	Dose & Route	Contraindications	Responsibilities During Administration	Potential Complications
Phenylephrine (Neosynephrine)				
• Relief of nasal congestion	**Adult:** • Administer intranasally • Give 2-3 gtts/spray of 0.25 – 0.5% solution in each nostril no more frequently than q 3-4 hrs • Or, give 2-3 gtts/spray of 1% solution in each nostril no more frequently than q 4h. **Pediatric:** • < 2 yrs – individualized by physician • 2-6 years: 2-3 gtts/0.125 or 0.16% solution q 4 hrs.PRN • 6 to 12 years: 2-3 gtts/sprays of 0.25% solution q 4 hrs PRN	• Use caution in patients with: - Cardiovascular disease - Hypertension - Diabetes mellitus - Hyperthyroidism - Hypersensitivity - C losed angle glaucoma	• Advise patient a mild, transient stinging sensation may occur after application • Rinse tip of dropper or spray bottle with hot water, dry and re-cap	• Headache • Lightheadedness • Nervousness • Rebound nasal congestion • Tachycardia • Trembling

Indications	Dose & Route	Contraindications	Responsibilities During Administration	Potential Complications
Photofrin				
• Reduction of obstruction and palliation of symptoms in patients with complete or partially obstructive non-small cell lung cancer	• 2 mg/kg • May be repeated up to three times, but injections must be separated by a minimum of 30 days	• Porphyria or known allergies to porphyrins • Patients with existing tracheoesophageal or bronchoesophageal fistula • Patient with tumors eroding into a major vessel • Patient with esophageal cancer eroding into the trachea • Patients with varices should be treated with extreme caution • Pregnant • Breast feeding	• Explain to patient the purpose and action of drug • Provide extensive education as outlined in procedure or drug insert prior to administration • Administer as a slow IV injection over 3-5 minutes • Reconstitute each vial with 31.8 ml of either 5% dextrose injection or 0.9 sodium chloride, to yield a final concentration of 2.5 mg/ml • Shake well until dissolved • Protect solution from bright light after mixing • Use immediately after reconstitution	• Light sensitivity post injection (see warnings) from the moment Photofrin is injected and for approximately 30 days thereafter, skin and eyes will be very sensitive to bright light • Exposure to bright or direct light will cause sunburn, redness and swelling • Itching

Indications	Dose & Route	Contraindications	Responsibilities During Administration	Potential Complications
Prochlorperazine (Compazine)				
• Control of severe nausea and vomiting • Short term treatment of generalized anxiety and agitation • Before anesthesia	**<u>Adult</u>** • 5 – 10 mg IV 15-30 minutes before and/or after anesthesia • IV infusion 20 mg per liter D_5W or normal saline 15-30 minutes before anesthesia • Not to exceed 40 mg per day **<u>Pediatric</u>** • Over 10 kg or > 2 years 0.1-0.15 mg/kg/dose IM • Not recommended for IV administration in children	• Comatose patient • Presence of large amounts of CNS depressants (alcohol, barbiturates, narcotics) • < 2 years old or < 20 pounds • Reyes syndrome or other encephalopathy	• Protect medication from light until ready to use • If markedly discolored, discard • Do not mix with any other agents except isotonic solutions if diluting • Do not give as a bolus; give slowly • Observe for abnormal movement • Dilute 5 mg with 0.9 ml of NS	• Neuroleptic malignant syndrome • Respiratory depression • Hyperpyrexia, muscle rigidity, altered mental status, tachycardia, irregular pulse, irregular blood pressure, cardiac dysrhythmias, diaphoresis • Tardive dyskinesia • Hypotension • Deep sleep to coma • Pseudo-Parkinson's disease • Non-specific ECG changes

Indications	Dose & Route	Contraindications	Responsibilities During Administration	Potential Complications
Promethazine (Phenergan)				
• For prevention and control of nausea and vomiting • As an adjunct to other sedative and analgesic medications	**Adult** • For sedation, 25-50 mg IV • For antiemetic, 12.5-25 mg q 4 h PRN **Pediatric** • 0.25-0.5 mg/kg/dose q 4-6 h prn • Do NOT use in children under 2 years of age	• Hypersensitivity to promethazine, penicillins or to sulfa drugs • Glaucoma • Comatose patient • < 2 years of age • Lower respiratory tract infection • Concurrent use of other CNS depressants • Pregnancy • Reyes Syndrome • Bone marrow • Depression • Acute asthma • Children with hepatic disease	• Do not give faster than 25 mg per minute • Administer through a port on IV line, not directly into vein • Reduce barbiturate dose by half if given simultaneously • Reduce dose in elderly patients, if possible • Administer with caution and carefully observe patients with history of prostatic hypertrophy, stenosing peptic ulcer, bladder neck obstruction, and pyloduodenal obstruction because of the anticholinergic effect	• Venous thrombosis at injection site • Neuroleptic malignant syndrome • Apnea in neonates, infants, and young children • Hallucinations • Seizures • Respiratory depression • Sudden death • Tachycardia • Bradycardia • Unconsciousness • Hypotension/ Hypertension • Phlebitis

Indications	Dose & Route	Contraindications	Responsibilities During Administration	Potential Complications
Racepinephrine Inhalation Solution USP, 2.25% (Racemic Epinephrine)				
• Temporary relief of shortness of breath, tightness of chest and wheezing • Reduces mucosal and submucosal edema • Reduces airway smooth muscle spasm	• IMPORTANT: DO NOT allow contact with metal • 0.5 ml (approximately 10 gtts) of solution into nebulizer reservoir. Add 3 ml of normal saline diluent. Gently swirl the nebulizer to mix contents. Administer for 15 minutes q 3-4 h	• Pregnancy • Nursing mother • MAO inhibitor drugs within past two weeks • Use with caution with - hypertension - heart disease - thyroid disease - diabetes - dysuria due to enlarged prostate gland - antidepressants - liver disease	• Protect medication from light until ready to use • Do not use if markedly discolored	• Tremors • Sleeplessness • Nausea • Loss of appetite • Rapid heart rate • Nervousness • Possible effects on the heart • Headache • Tachycardia

References

American Society and Health System. (2010). Pharmacists Drug Information. Retrieved on Jan 27, 2012 at www.ahfsdruginformation.com.

Medline Plus; US National Library of Medicine. National Institute of Health 2012. Retrieved on Jan 21, 2012 at www.nlm.nih.gov/medlineplus/druginfo.

Skidmore Roth, L. (2011). *Nursing drug reference*. St. Louis: Mosby.

Society of Gastroenterology Nurses and Associates, Inc. (2008). *Gastroenterology Nursing: A Core Curriculum*. Chicago, IL: Author.

Thomson Reuters. (2012). Micromedex Formulary Advisor. Montvale, NJ: Thomson Reuters Healthcare.

Thomson Reuters. (2009). *Physicians Desk Reference Nurses Drug Handbook*. Montvale, NJ: Thomson Reuters Healthcare.

Appendix B

Special Considerations for Bronchoscopy in the Mechanically Ventilated Patient

[Use in conjunction with Flexible Bronchoscopy, page 1]

Flexible bronchoscopy can be performed in almost any extremely ill patient. Bronchoscopy has become an indispensable tool in the optimal management of intensive care patients with both diagnostic and therapeutic goals. It has been increasingly done on mechanically-ventilated patients. Mechanically-ventilated patients are predisposed to increased risk of complications and as a result bronchoscopy must be done by very skilled personnel.

Increased Risks

The potential high-risk patients will be those with:

1. Significant hypoxemia
2. Bleeding diathesis
3. Recent acute myocardial infarction
4. Intractable dysrhythmias
5. Cardiovascular instability requiring vasopressor support
6. Uncontrolled bronchospasm
7. High baseline peak airway pressures
8. Significant auto PEEP $\geq$ 15 cm H_2O
9. Severe cranial hypertension syndrome
10. Known CO_2 retainers

Possible Alterations in Pulmonary Mechanics and Gas Exchange

Because of the highly technical nature of modern ventilator equipment and the need to make moment-to-moment adjustments based on the patient's response during the procedure, it is necessary that an appropriately skilled individual (e.g., Respiratory Therapist) be present during the procedure to address these unique aspects.

In the intubated and mechanically ventilated patient flexible bronchoscopy causes temporary alterations of respiratory mechanics related to the increased airway resistance produced by the bronchoscope. Areas of consideration during the procedure include:

1. During volume controlled ventilation, the preset pressure limit may prevent the desired volume from being delivered.
2. The delivered respiratory gases can be lost through leaks in the adapters used to accommodate the procedure.
3. Suctioning through the bronchoscope will decrease the tidal volume being delivered.
4. PEEP baseline may dramatically decrease or increase.
5. Reductions in lung volume and functional residual capacity may produce alveolar closure.
6. Reflex bronchospasm may be induced by stimulation of vagal receptors in the upper airway.
7. Expiratory flow is impeded and the duration of expiration may be insufficient to allow the lung to deflate.

Complications

1. Same as Flexible Bronchoscopy
2. Severe arterial oxygen desaturations
3. Pneumothorax and barotrauma
4. Ventricular tachycardia

5. Bradycardia

Technical Considerations During Flexible Bronchoscopy

1. The outside diameter of the flexible bronchoscope in relation to the internal diameter of the endotracheal tube is the first aspect to consider. A 5 mm outside diameter bronchoscope occupies 30% of the cross sectional area of a 9 mm internal diameter endotracheal tube, 40% of an 8 mm and about 50% of a 7mm. If a standard size bronchoscope is used most authors recommend that the ET tube should be at least 8 mm in internal diameter.
2. A bite block should be used to prevent damage to the endoscope and/or endotracheal tube.
3. A swivel adapter is attached to the endotracheal tube.
4. If short-acting paralytic agents are used to reduce the risk of barotrauma and to prevent cough and "fighting" the ventilator during the procedure, sedatives should also be administered. Renal status should be checked before giving short-acting paralytic agents.
5. An appropriately credentialed individual must address the following measures:
    a. Prior to initiating the procedure the patient is ventilated with the following suggested ventilator settings:
        1) volume controlled ventilation.
        2) FIO2 100%.
        3) peak inspiratory flow lower than 60 l/m.
        4) withdrawal of PEEP if it is being employed.
        5) peak pressure alarm titrated to a level that allows adequate ventilation.
    b. During the procedure, monitor patient response and adjust ventilatory parameters as needed.
        1) Monitor tidal volume.
        2) Keep expired volumes as close as possible to pre-bronchoscopic values and to avoid excessive levels of auto-PEEP.
6. At the end of the procedure:
    a. FIO_2 is reduced to appropriate levels to maintain oxygen saturation per order.
    b. Other modified ventilator modifications returned to pre-procedure settings as patient condition warrants.
    c. Chest X-ray is recommended to rule out barotrauma or pneumothorax.

References

Anzueto, A., Levine, S. M., & Jenkinson, S. G. (1992). The technique of fiberoptic bronchoscopy. Diagnostic and therapeutic uses in intubated, ventilated patients. *Journal of Critical Illness, 7,:* 1657-1664.

Dettenmier, P. A. (1992). *Pulmonary nursing care* (pp.331-369). St. Louis: Mosby-Year Book.

Jolliet, P. H., & Chevrolet, J. C. (1992). Bronchoscopy in the intensive care unit. *Intensive Care Medicine,* 18, 160-169.

Raoof, S., Mehrishi, S. & Prakash, UB. (2001). Role of bronchoscopy in modern medical intensive care unit. *Clinics in Chest Medicine*, 22(2), 241-261.

Rodriguez de Castro, F., & Sole, J. (1996). Flexible bronchoscopy in mechanically ventilated patients. *Journal of Bronchology, 3,* 64-68.

Tai, D. Y. (1998). Bronchoscopy in the intensive care unit. *Annals of the Academy of Medicine of Singapore, 27,* 552.

Appendix C

Oxygen Therapy for the Patient Undergoing a Pulmonary Procedure

For the patient requiring supplemental oxygen an appropriate delivery device should be chosen based on the patient's condition. Each device has different characteristics. These delivery devices provide low flow, low concentration or higher flow, higher concentration. Ability of end-tidal CO_2 monitoring should be anticipated.

Methods of Oxygen Delivery

1. Nasal cannula or nasal prongs - deliver low concentrations of oxygen. The prongs permit talking, eating and suctioning without removal. The inspired oxygen concentration depends on the flow of oxygen. For every liter per minute increase, the inspired oxygen concentration will increase by approximately 4%. Oxygen used with a nasal cannula with a flow of 1-6 liters per minute is 24% to 44% concentration. This system is acceptable for patients with minimal or no respiratory distress.
2. Face mask - If a mask is used to deliver the oxygen, it is important to make sure the flow rate is at least 5 liters per minute. The recommended flow is 8 to 10 liters per minute. These flows will allow the mask to be flushed and not collect exhaled carbon dioxide. This system can provide oxygen concentrations as high as 40% to 60%.
   Note that the crudeness of the simple mask makes it impossible to predict exact oxygen concentration.
3. Face mask with oxygen reservoir - This system has constant flow of oxygen into an attached reservoir, which may provide oxygen concentrations higher than 60%. A flow of 6 l/m will provide this concentration and each liter per minute increase in flow will increase the inspired oxygen concentration by 10%. When this mask is used properly, at 10 l/m the oxygen concentration is almost 100%.
   This mask system is most appropriate for spontaneously breathing patients who require the highest possible oxygen concentrations.
4. Venturi mask - The Venturi mask provides a high gas flow but with a more fixed oxygen concentration. Oxygen under pressure is passed through a narrow orifice and after leaving the orifice, provides a subatmospheric pressure that entrains room air into the system. The oxygen concentration is adjusted by changing the orifice and oxygen flow.
   Note that there are many varieties of this style of mask.
   Typically with the Venturi mask, oxygen delivery concentrations may be adjusted to 24%, 28%, 35% and 40%.

Never withhold oxygen from patients who have respiratory distress simply because you may suspect hypoxic ventilatory drive.

Mode of Delivery	O_2 Concentration	Advantages	Disadvantages	Possible Complications
Nasal Cannula/Nasal Prongs	Flow of 1-6 liters per minute is 24% - 44% concentration	• Easy to apply • Light • Allows patient mobility • Talking, eating and suctioning possible	• Easily dislodged • Nares dryness and bleeding • Skin breakdown around ears	

Appendix C

<table>
<tr><td>Face Mask</td><td>Concentrations of 35% - 60%</td><td></td><td rowspan="3">• Uncomfortable and hot
• Irritation of skin caused by tight fit
• Difficult to control FIO_2
• Must be removed to eat</td><td rowspan="3">• Patients who are prone to vomit may aspirate
• May cause CO_2 retention and hypoventilation if flow is too low and exhalation ports are obstructed</td></tr>
<tr><td>Face Mask with Reservoir
• Partial re-breathing
• Non-re-breathing</td><td>• Concentrations of 35% - 60%
• Concentrations of 90% or greater</td><td>• Ideal method for delivering high O_2 concentration for short-term purposes</td></tr>
<tr><td>Venturi Mask</td><td>• Adjustments allow for delivery of precise O_2 concentrations of 24% - 40%</td><td>• Best suited for patient who must have a consistent FIO_2</td></tr>
</table>

Potential Complications

1. With PaO_2 >60 torr, ventilatory depression may occur in spontaneously breathing patients with elevated $PaCO_2$.
2. With FIO_2 >0.5, absorption atelectasis, oxygen toxicity, and/or depression of ciliary and/or leukocytic function may occur.
3. Supplemental oxygen should be administered with caution to patients suffering from paraquat poisoning and to patients receiving bleomycin.
4. Fire hazard is increased in the presence of increased oxygen concentrations.

References

Aspach, J. G. (Ed.). (2006). *Core curriculum for critical care nurses* (6th ed.) Philadelphia: Saunders.
Dettenmeier, P. A. (1992). *Pulmonary nursing care.* St. Louis: Mosby-Year Book.
Zevitz, M., Plantz, S., & Gossman, W. (2006). *Advanced Cardiac Life Support (ACLS).* New York: McGraw-Hill Companies.

GLOSSARY

Glossary

-A-

acid/base disorders, metabolic: abnormal pH of body fluids resulting from altered acid production (other than carbonic acid)

acid/base disorders, respiratory: abnormal pH of body fluids resulting from altered elimination of carbon dioxide

airways, lower: structures that also conduct air to and from the lung parenchyma; lined with ciliated mucus membranes that sweep and remove excess mucus and debris to be coughed out of the respiratory tract. Include trachea, tracheobronchial tree, mainstem bronchi, bronchioles.

airways, upper: structures that serve as filters and passageways for air being inspired and expired; airways warm and moisten inhaled air and provide the protective reflexes of sneezing and the closing of the larynx to prevent aspiration. Include nose, mouth, pharynx and larynx.

Allen test: test for collateral blood flow between radial and ulnar arteries. Digital compression of both ulnar and radial arteries causes palmar blanching followed by hyperemia when either artery is released.

aliquots: a portion that represents a known quantity; one of several quantities of the same size.

argon plasma coagulation: a method of producing hemostasis and tissue devitalization using a stream of argon gas in a specialized non-contact monopolar electrosurgical unit.

atelectasis: a collapsed or airless condition of the lung or a portion thereof.

-B-

bag-valve-mask resuscitator: manually-operated resuscitator consisting of a bag reservoir, a one-way flow valve, and a face mask capable of ventilating a non-breathing patient. Commonly known as an Ambu™ bag.

barotrauma: injury caused by a change in atmospheric pressure between a potentially closed space and the surrounding area.

biopsy, endobronchial: taking small tissue samples from the airway using a biopsy forceps.

biopsy forceps, hot: electrocoagulating forceps used to obtain tissue samples when the patient is at an increased risk of bleeding.

biopsy, transbronchial: taking small tissue samples from the lung parenchyma using a biopsy forceps.

bipolar electrocoagulation: an electrocoagulation method in which the electrical current flows between two small electrodes on the tip of the probe, both of which are in contact with the target tissue

blood gas analysis: chemical analysis of the blood for concentration of oxygen and carbon dioxide.

brachytherapy, intrabronchial: involves the placement of a flexible, small-caliber afterloading catheter into or near a tumor via direct visual guidance of a bronchoscope.

broncholith: a calculus in the bronchus.

bronchoscope: an endoscope designed to pass through the trachea to allow visual inspection of the tracheobronchial tree; also designed to permit the passage of an instrument that can be used to obtain tissue for biopsy or to remove a foreign body from the tracheobronchial tree.

bronchoscopy: the direct endoscopic visualization and examination of the trachea and the tracheobronchial tree using a flexible bronchoscope.

bronchospasm: abnormal narrowing with obstruction of the lumen of the bronchi due to spasm of the peribronchial smooth muscle.

brushing: using a cytology brush to obtain samples of the respiratory mucosa for microscopic examination.

-C-

capacity: the amount of air contained in the lung at a defined phase of respiration. Same as **volume**.

chyle: milk-like, alkaline contents of the lacteals and lymphatic vessels of the intestine, consisting of the products of digestion and principally absorbed fats.

chylothorax: chyle in the pleural cavities.

cryotherapy: exposing tissues to extreme cold in order to produce well-demarcated areas of cell injury and destruction.

-D-

devitalization: destruction or loss of vitality.

diathesis: constitutional predisposition to certain disease conditions.

diffusion: the exchange of air from and to the blood/gas barrier (alveolar-capillary exchange)

-E-

embolism, air: air bubble in the veins, right atrium or ventricle, or capillaries.

emphysema, subcutaneous: presence of air in the subcutaneous tissue.

empyema: pus in a body cavity, esp. in the pleural cavity (pyothorax).

expiratory reserve volume (ERV): the maximum volume of air that can be exhaled from the resting end-expiratory level.

-F-

FiO_2: fraction of inspired oxygen; expressed as the percentage of inspired air composed of oxygen.

fluid, exudative: pleural fluid that has a high protein content; is often opaque and may indicate pneumonia (parapneumonic effusion), tuberculosis, or other pulmonary infection.

fluid, pleural: serous secretion that lubricates the potential space between the visceral and parietal pleura, reducing friction during respiratory movements of the lung.

fluid, transudative: pleural fluid that is usually clear; has a low protein content; and is often associated with congestive heart failure, cirrhosis or renal failure (also called serous).

fulguration: destruction of tissue by means of high-frequency electric sparks.

functional residual capacity (FRC): the volume of air remaining in the lungs at the resting end-expiratory level. FRC = ERV+ RV

-H-

hemothorax: blood or body fluid in the pleural cavity caused by rupture of blood vessels.

hypertension, pulmonary: increase in blood pressure through the pulmonary system; alveolar hypoxia is the most important causative mechanism, which results either from localized inadequate ventilation of alveoli that are well-perfused or from a generalized decrease in alveolar ventilation.

hypoventilation: reduced rate and depth of breathing.

hypoxemia: insufficient oxygenation of the blood.
hypoxemia, refractory: hypoxemia which does not respond to usual treatment.

-I-

inspiratory capacity (IC): the maximum volume of air that can be inhaled from the normal resting end-expiratory level. $IC = V_T + IRV$

inspiratory reserve volume (IRV): the maximum volume of air that can be inhaled following and above a normal tidal inspiration.

-L-

laryngospasm: spasm of the laryngeal muscles.

lavage, bronchoalveolar: flooding a pulmonary subsegment with sterile non-bacteriostatic saline and suctioning the instilled fluid; the material obtained is then sent for cytologic, microbiologic, and/or chemical analysis.

-M-

mediastinal shift: displacement of the mediastinal structures caused by pneumothorax; detectable as cardiac dullness and apex beat shifted away from the affected side.

methemoglobinemia: clinical condition in which more than 1% of hemoglobin in the blood has been oxidized to the ferric (Fe^{+++}) form; principal sign is cyanosis, because the oxidized hemoglobin is incapable of transporting oxygen. May result from a reaction to local anesthetics, among other causes.

monopolar electrocoagulation: an electrocoagulation method in which the electrical current flows between a small, active electrode that is in contact with the target tissue and a larger grounding pad that is attached to the patient's skin.

mucopurulent: contains pus and exudate.

-N-

nebulizer: an apparatus for producing a fine spray or mist.

-P-

parenchyma: structures where actual gas exchange occurs. Alveolar ducts, alveolar sacs.

PaO_2: partial pressure of oxygen dissolved in arterial blood.

$PaCO_2$: partial pressure of carbon dioxide dissolved in arterial blood.

PCO_2: partial pressure of carbon dioxide.

PEEP: positive end-expiratory pressure; used in intubated patients with respiratory failure; increases mean alveolar pressure to re-open closed alveolar units.

perfusion: the movement of blood to and from the capillary bed.

pH: potential of Hydrogen; the degree of acidity or alkalinity of a substance.

photodynamic therapy: method of targeting and destroying cancer cells while sparing surrounding healthy tissue; two-step process involving administration of a photoactive drug, then exposing the cancerous tissue to a specific frequency of laser light.

photosensitivity: condition in which the skin reacts abnormally to light, especially ultraviolet radiation or sunlight.

pleura: serous membrane that covers the exterior of both lungs (visceral pleura) and is reflected upon the walls of the thorax and diaphragm (parietal pleura).

pneumothorax: a collection of air or gas in the pleural cavity.

pO_2: partial pressure of oxygen.

porphyria: a hereditary or acquired enzyme defect in which the biosynthesis of heme, in either the bone marrow or liver, leads to an overproduction of porphyrins or their precursors; two cardinal symptoms are photosensitivity and neurologic disturbances.

proteinosis, alveolar: accumulation of excess protein in the alveoli.

purulent: filled with pus; indicates infection.

-R-

residual volume (RV): the volume of air that remains in the lungs following a maximum expiration.

-S-

serosanguinous: bloody; in pleural fluid, may indicate the presence of malignancy.

space, pleural: the potential space between the visceral and parietal pleura.

stent: self-expanding stainless steel mesh device introduced into a lumen (e.g., coronary artery, pulmonary airway, biliary duct) to prevent lumen closure.

stridor: a musical sound, audible without a stethoscope, and predominantly inspiratory.

syringe, heparinized: a syringe in which a small volume of heparin solution is used to coat the interior of the barrel for the purpose of preventing the blood sample from clotting.

-T-

thoracostomy: resection of the chest wall to allow drainage of the chest cavity.

tidal volume (V_T): the volume of air that is inhaled and exhaled with each normal breath.

torr: 1 mm Hg

total lung capacity (TLC): the volume of air contained within the lungs following a maximum inspiration. TLC = IRV + V_T + ERV + RV or TLC = IC + FRC or TLC = VC + RV

transducer: device that converts one form of energy to another; used in medical electronics to receive the energy produced by sound or pressure and relay it as an electrical impulse to another transducer which can either convert the energy back into its original form or make a record of it on a recording device.

-U-

ultrasound, endobronchial: uses an ultrasound probe through a bronchoscope to image the bronchial tree and adjacent structures.

-V-

vasopressor: an agent that stimulates contraction of the muscles of capillaries and arteries, increasing resistance to blood flow and elevating blood pressure.

ventilation: the exchange of air from the environment to the lungs.

ventilation, volume controlled: mechanically-assisted ventilation in which the volume of air delivered is set and the pressure varies.

vital capacity (VC): the maximum volume of air that may be exhaled following a maximum inspiration or inhaled following a maximum expiration. VC = IRV + V_T + ERV or VC = IC + ERV

volume: the amount of air contained in the lung at a defined phase of respirations. Same as **capacity**.

Index